INTIMATE ENCOUNTERS

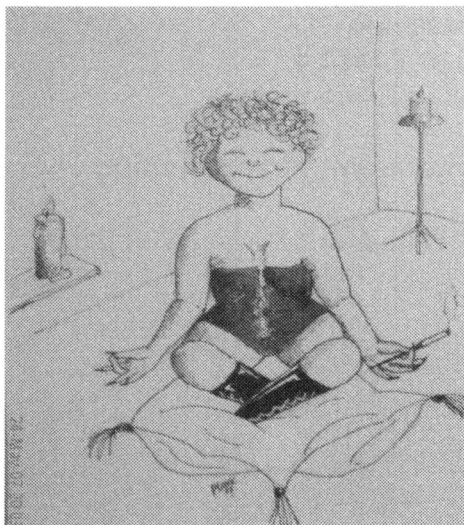

By Rose Budworth Levine

One million people commit suicide every year.'
the World Health Organization

Rose Budworth Levine

Published by
Chipmunkapublishing
PO Box 6872
Brentwood
Essex CM13 1ZT
United Kingdom

http://www.chipmunkapublishing.com

INTIMATE ENCOUNTERS

DEDICATION

Rose Budworth Levine

INTIMATE ENCOUNTERS

Dedication

It's been one of those manic weeks; everything has got on top of me. I have wanted to run. That's what I always want to do when everything gets just too much. It would be easier to stay in bed, not to work, not pay the bills, to just give up. It's been a strange week. I have finished with my boyfriend, well, at least for now. I have been crying all week. I try not to put my book off any longer. I receive a call from my publisher, which has given me the momentum to finish it. I have working all week, it feels like all of my life has been wrapped up tying up lose ends like a chapter in my life has finished waiting for the next one to start.

It's interesting that we push the one person we love the most away in times of crisis or maybe its just circumstance. Who knows why we do things. All I know is I am glad my book is finished. I have talked about my book to everyone and shown it to only a few of my closest friends. Yet, the most important person that needs to read it is the person I now dedicate my book to. It's the one person who has never judged me, has accepted me for who I am. He is one of my best friends, my lover and soul mate, the person that's knows me best, my boyfriend Jamie.

Rose Budworth Levine

INTIMATE ENCOUNTERS

1- THE SINS OF THE FATHERS

Where does one start to write a book about a lifetime full of promises and adventure, and where the heartaches bleed you dry, and where because of your lost innocence as a child you end up subconsciously as an adult with the driving ambition for an alternative lifestyle? A lifestyle, which takes you on an emotional roller coaster, that last for months and years of your life, and me a woman of wanton love lust and desire.

A journey that entwines and encompasses some of the magical mysteries of the human flesh and the physical needs of both species, but leaves you none the wiser, as to what makes the species tick emotionally and sexually.

A journey that brings smiles, laughter, excitement, fear and the many tears that scars and wounds you deeply from the gathering pace of relationships that come and go in your tumultuous life. One that peels and exposes your inner self, layer by layer, as you continually feel the exhilaration and the pumping heartbeats pounding your breasts, as with each touch of a hand or caress on your flesh you feel vulnerable, naked and confused even scared, as a new pulsating man climbs abroad your waiting torso, without any thought to my sensitivity, my feelings and my desires of wanting to be loved. He smiles, he looks, he wants to run and hide, he says, 'I'll see you around' as he leaves my side. What more

7

can I do, I am female, I am capable of taking the next, and the next, and the next man in succession, but always they deliver the same coldness, as they pries your virtues from you and leave with there dignity limp, shrivelled and rather forlorn for the five banging minutes they have given me. So what the hell does all this tell me as a woman, what does this mean for man., as at the end, he leaves you with a spent force and you empty inside, and left wondering whether you are even sane and of the same human species, are there any normal men out there, are any capable of loving me a woman, a complex woman such as I. It may have began with a look, a touch and a few silly words that made us lie together or could it have been the alcohol or could it have been me who was the romantic, as his hand felt my knee and wandered up my thigh under the hem of my dress. Only the reader can decide for him or herself, but can you decide, are you just as confused as me with your relationship that began with your passions all aflame and burning brightly as you kissed?

Well I suppose I should begin with me, who am I? My name is Rose Budworth-Levine and if you believe that you believe anything. I am a born fantasist and romantic and despite my persona I believe in Karma, I believe in the tooth fairy and I believe in prince charming even though I met and married a couple of frogs along the way. I was born about forty years ago, give or take a couple of years and was raised and bought up in the South of England along with my two brothers and working class parents. I always thought of my childhood as being pretty normal apart from being singled out from an early age as a gifted child and being on the plump side. But perhaps as his story unfolds it wasn't quite as normal as most.

My parents were to divorce late later in life. They stuck it out for nearly 35 years. I am not sure whether my mother deserved a medal for that or a certificate in stupidity and ignorance. All I know is our childhood upbringing helps to mould our future. All families have their little secrets, and I do not blame my parents for my quirky little habits but there are some things we need to keep private from our children and one of them is our bedroom secrets which is why I have written this book anonymously, I don't really want my daughter reading them.

So lets start with my mother who was a very attractive woman, with the figure of Sophia Loren; well that's how I remember her. She was bought up from a working class family her father worked for the same firm all of his life. She was a churchgoer and had the voice of an angel. She had been chosen to be an opera singer quite young but her parents could not afford to send her to Switzerland so she never realized her ambitions and then her mother was struck down with multiple sclerosis when my mother was in her teens so she had to care of for her younger sister. We all have dreams and my mother is no different from the rest of us. She wanted to be a draughtswoman, she was a gifted painter but her uncle who worked for a well-known razor blade company suggested that being a draughtswoman was not a woman's job. So she left home at 19 when she met my father. She was clever, resourceful and spent her time at home with all of us; she worked hard at being a good parent, and teaching us the joys of macramé, painting and anything else that came to mind. She took part time jobs in between looking after us to make ends meat. She was patient and a skilled dressmaker who taught me how to sew at the age of seven. I could make my own clothes by the time I was a teenager.

On the downside she suffered from ill health and severe depression and would take to her bed for long periods at a time ranging from a few hours to a few days and we as children worried relentlessly over her state of health. Our home life was pretty chaotic we lived in various different parts of the country depending where dad decided to move to. I think we moved about 7 times during my childhood. My father always wanted to do different things he had so many different business, that would often fail and then we would have to move house. We lived in a pub. We lived in a wonderful house with acres of land and then we were off again on a whim. That's just what we did. Our house was always lively with lots of visitors. It was either clean or tidy or a total mess. Mum would spend days in bed being depressed or having a "bad back" and when we did have visitors it was all panic and hands on to clean the place up the day before so that everyone would come round and see that the house was normal.

My father always said he never knew what mood my mum was going to be in when he got home, whether she would be happy or depressed. She was so gifted, on her good days she would paint and draw, redecorate the house from top to bottom and on her bad days she would stay in bed and wallow in her depression and then tell us kids all about it. I guess my dad didn't help much but I will come to him later. My mum was very "open" if that's the word I am looking for always telling me in graphic detail about her sex life with my dad. Not that I really wanted to know that at twelve years old or telling me how small his Willy was. I think it was her way of punishing him for his misdemeanours.

So let's move onto my dad, my father was also an attractive man, with the personality of the eternal optimist. His father was an alcoholic and his mother was a bit of a slapper I suppose. She use to have to raid his pockets to feed the kids and from all accounts use to send little Jackie down the shops for sweets while she entertained the latest boyfriend. I hated his father, he used to come and visit us when we were kids. He was very creepy and used to come over and stay with us and usually chuck up all over my bedroom floor after he had had a few too many to drink on a Sunday afternoon. Luckily it wasn't very often only every couple of years. He didn't like the boys in the family very much only liked little girls which as an adult is pretty worrying but then there was always a bit of history of incest in my dads side of the family. Not that my dad was like that not at all, he was kind and loving and a great father, I remember my eldest brother joining the boy scouts once and my dad took him out after a couple of weeks because he had been interfered with himself when he was younger and he wasn't having anything happen to his sons. He was the most hard workingman I have ever known along with my ex husband. He was made redundant more times that any many I know. Worked in the car trade and would bounce back each time and go out and get another job. I think in all the years he worked he was only unemployed for 3 weeks.

My father never wanted to be like his own dad, have his mum always raiding his pockets when he was drunk to pay for food. Buying presents for my dad and then taking them back, or pawning them out because he needed the money again. I remember him telling me a story about a piano where his dad had bought him this lovely piano and then taken it back a couple of weeks later. But he was the kind of person that would make promises he couldn't always keep and I hated that.

He was a charmer, always wanting to play the part of the good guy, but sadly he was a compulsive womanizer, and my mother well she was just walking around with rose coloured blinkers on. I told her as a teenager why do you stay with my dad all these years and put up with his affairs and she would say, "because I love him". I remember the break-ups, the reconciliation's, and the attempted suicide on my father's part when one day my mother did finally kick him out. Of course she took him back. I remember my mother's nervous breakdown after the birth of my youngest brother and how all in all it had a huge impact on our lives and still haunts us today as adults and parents.

During my fathers relationships with other woman, most of which I knew about, either from his body language, or the way in which he flirted with particular women. My mother had had a couple of affairs, I guess to pay my father back for his womanizing, however one of them was a teacher I had been dating. Not a teacher at my school but a friend of my brother Sean. He was much older than me and I guess I had a teenage crush on him. I found out that my mother had been having an affair with him. When I confronted her she said he made her feel good about herself and I think she dismissed my infatuation with him because I had not had sex and said she was unaware that I was seeing him. I felt like my whole trust in my mother was shattered.

My father's behaviour had a terrible effect on my mother she suffered from low self-esteem and time again not knowing which of her best friends my father was going to take to bed and fuck. The manipulation and lies played havoc with my mothers' head. Deep down I think she knew all the time when he was having affairs because I always did. But when she would confront him he would say she was crazy or depressed and wasn't it about time she went back to the doctors and went on the anti depressants again.   None of it was done in a violent way, all very underhand, but I knew everything and that was half the problem.

My mother had this romantic idea that all marriages could be like her own parents, they had been married until the day they died. Met as teenagers and although poor, they seemed happy with what little they had. My grandfather suffered with ulcers for years whilst my grandmother looked after him but then she developed multiple sclerosis at the age of thirty, my grandfather looked after her for the rest of his life. One day he died of a heart attack whilst buying a packet of tampax for my auntie who was visiting my grandmother who was ill at the time in hospital. She died three months later. My mum always said later she died of a broken heart as she had lost the will to fight after that. I was 23 when she died. One week before my wedding. How I miss my grandparents.

INTIMATE ENCOUNTERS

2 - I WANT TO BE A PRINCESS

Now let's move onto the rest of my family. I am the middle of two brothers my eldest was always the golden boy. His name was Sean. He was tall dark, handsome and very charming. He was the type of person no one could dislike and had girls falling at his feet, he even managed to work his way through and date all of my girlfriends at school. I loved him to bits and always wished I could meet a man like my brother, Sean. He was always much focused on what he wanted to do in life, unlike me "Miss Scatty Brain" that could do anything but didn't have a clue what she wanted in life. He used to joke and say he was going to grow up and become a gigolo but he wanted to be a graphic designer from the age of seven and he wanted to live in America. He wanted to drive a Porsche and he wanted to have loads of money.

I on the other hand wanted to be a spy, and then I wanted to be a potter and then I wanted to be this and that. I changed with the wind. I never really knew what I wanted to do. I would dream about having five children all different nationalities, one half black, one half Chinese, one half middle east, one redhead, and one Italian. Instead I would enact out my fantasies adopting stray cats in the chicken coups in the large half acre garden we had during our childhood. I nurtured the cats and then when my mum found them and begged to keep them as I had been secretly feeding them for weeks. She would pay any vets bills if they were sick and then get them neutered and then they would get run over a couple of weeks later. I can't remember how many cats I have had over the years. My mother used to say it was my motherly instinct taking over being transferred to my animals, which became apparent when I was married years later with five cats having been told I could not have any children. Each one a different colour, one ginger, one black, one black and white, one white, one tabby.

When I was seven years old along came my younger brother John. It was a very difficult time then; I don't remember too much I think our brains have a way of blocking out traumatic times during our childhood. My mother went into labour early but I was told afterwards that my father had had an affair during the pregnancy, yet again. When he told her it must have triggered her into an early labour. He was so pathetic and insensitive he even took his girlfriend into the hospital just after my mother had given birth in the hospital. It was one of my mums "best friends". She came home about 4 weeks later with the baby and I don't remember much at all for the next few months apart from lots of visits from my second mum my auntie Beth, her sister and lots of helping around the house. I used to do lots of housework when I was small I remember my mum saying to me I could run a house and look after my brother, John standing on my head at eleven. Not surprising really. Mum felt like she would never be able to cope without my father so needless to say mum took dad back again and again and again.

INTIMATE ENCOUNTERS

My eldest brother Sean once said he wanted to run away from the family and move abroad because my mother was so difficult to handle and he had little respect for my father. It affected my younger brother John far more severely; he was living with my mother towards the end of the marriage. Both my brother Sean and I had married and moved away by then. He slipped into a life and drugs and self harming after they split up and then left and married a woman many years older than him, and he abandoned the family altogether and still lives in total denial and once had a breakdown during his adult life.

How it affected me, well it is far too complex for me to even comprehend. Years of counselling have helped me. I guess I should be more pissed at my dad but in some ways I was more pissed at my mum for putting up with all his womanizing. I knew if I ever married I would never let a man be unfaithful to me.

I remember a time when I was to feel totally devastated by my mothers' actions. I went out for the evening with some friends. We were about thirteen and I always looked and dressed much older than my years. We were sitting in a pub having orange juice and chatting when a man that I recognized from a few years before came up to me. He had been a customer as my parents had previously run a pub. He had a friend called Ian who used to take both my brothers and me out with him to stock car racing. I had a huge crush on him and liked the way he made me feel. He always used to say how pretty I was and how grown up I looked and I would look forward to our time together as my father was always busy running the business.

His friend came over to me and said hello and asked me how my parents were. I told him they were fine since selling the pub and then he bought up the subject of my mother. He said "You remember your mother used too go to the beauty parlour every Wednesday". I smiled and said I remembered it well. Then he replied, "Well she never went to the beauty parlour she was off shagging Ian". My friends who had overheard looked at me, the tears started to flow down my cheeks and I got up from where I was sitting and went into the ladies room and cried and cried. I felt so humiliated and betrayed. How could my mother do such a thing? I confronted her again but she never really understood how I felt. I guess it was around that time that I stopped taking my male friends back to the house to meet my mother. She was always very flirtatious and because she was so attractive I felt like she would try and take them away from me again.

As for me well I am not quite sure what impact it had on my life. I know I never wanted to end up like my mother and I never wanted to marry a man like my father. I made a conscious decision not to get married early and to have children early. All of my friends at school had kids by the time they were 20. I wasn't married until I was 23 and had my first child at 28. I never wanted a daughter should I ever have one to grow up and feel threatened by their mothers sexuality in their teens. If I had a son I was going to bring them up to respect women and not be a cheating womanizer. As for me as much as we try to avoid being like our parents unfortunately history usually repeats itself and I guess I have been guilty of both at some point in my life, so perhaps in a peculiar way, my early years of family life did in fact change my life for the adventure I sought and experienced in later life.

During my early teenage years I was always curious about sex. Maybe it was because my parents fault or my mothers for describing how small his penis was and how she never really enjoyed sex with him. Or maybe it was because I found my mothers vibrator in the cupboard and pornographic magazines belonging to my father. Maybe it was because I just knew too much too soon and lost my innocence or maybe I was always going to be a sexually adventurous woman. One thing I have learnt through my journey of sexuality is I have no hang-ups about sex, I am not plagued by guilt nor do I blame my parents anymore. It just is.

I remember I was by chance searching through my parent's wardrobe looking for Christmas presents and I was about eleven years old at the time. I had always been a nosey child wanting to know the ins and outs of a cats arse. I was always asking questions and always searching for answers. I would always look for presents and then carefully unwrap them so that I could see what mum and dad had bought for Christmas. Then I would stick the tape back and hope no one would notice. My brother was older than me and I was about four and he was seven and I told him that Father Christmas didn't exist. I said mum and dad come in and bring in the presents and I remember he cried for days and went and told my mum and I got a smack.

So there I was at eleven being nosey again and found this black plastic bag tucked away at the back of the cupboard and out of curiosity I opened it and saw inside, I delved my hand into the bag and removed some Polaroid photographs of my mother naked on the bed. I couldn't believe there were pictures of my mum in the nude! Blimey is that what mum and dad do when they are in bed. I picked up was I realized now was a vibrating egg. It had a strange smell about it and I could not fathom what it was. It was an egg attached to a battery pack. As I turned the dial the egg started to vibrate in my hand. I could feel a strange sensation in my pussy and I placed the egg onto the outer lips of my pussy and felt it tingle. I started to feel wet and gently pushed the egg into my pussy and felt my whole body tingle as I turned up the dials and then down again. was excited and the feeling of this large object in my pussy was sent my whole body into my first orgasm, the sudden warm flush. I removed the egg and wiped it with some tissue and placed it back in the bag along with the magazines and pictures.

I felt slightly disgusted that something like that had made me feel so excited and I never masturbated again until I was nearly thirty-eight. I

INTIMATE ENCOUNTERS

guess it's all those taboos about sex and masturbation making your feel dirty. Boys have to listen to it all the time, especially if they come from a church going background. Stupid stories like if you wank or play with your cock it will drop off. Victorian attitudes leave people feeling isolated and ashamed. That's part of the problem people wanting to beat themselves up and feeling guilty and ashamed about their sexuality. Not me, I decided after my divorce I was going to explore myself fully and stop denying who I was. And this is where my story really begins

My first proper sexual experience was at thirteen. I had been seeing a man who was nineteen. We were going out for a few weeks and we used to kiss and fumble. All the usually things that teenagers do then one day he was kissing me goodnight and he asked me to give him oral sex or a "blow job" as he put it. We were on the porch way outside his parent's house, which was secluded from the street. I didn't know what to do. I didn't feel humiliated but I was curious so I got down on my knees and started to unzip his trousers. I did not play with his cock, which was semi-hard, but I took it in my mouth immediately. I started to suck the top and felt his cock become hard in my mouth. Within minutes his hand reached down and he took my hand and placed it on his cock on my hand and started to wank himself. I don't remember much apart from thinking how seedy it was but that I was keen to try "sex" again.

Rose Budworth Levine

I was thirteen when I was taken by what most people would now consider to be a paedophile. He was 40 years old and hung around with the group of people we went out with. I looked much older than my years. I could get into the local rugby club at 13 whilst the other girls much other had to provide ID. I was introduced to this man an attractive Irish man and he invited me over to his house. His name was Fred West, which was a bit worrying in hindsight and I don't remember much but him removing my knickers pushing me down on the bed and spread my legs and licked my pussy for hours. I don't even know if I struggled. He didn't try and have sex with me, I do remember that much. But as for seeing him again it was a nervy look from him when I was down the pub with the usual crowd known as "rent a crowd" as we used to go to parties together. Him arm in arm with his girlfriend who was about fifteen years older than me.

The first time I fell in love was with a man called David. He was twenty-one and I was nearly fourteen. I used to go to the local rugby club discos on a Saturday night. All the players would congregate in the bar at one end whilst guests would dance the night away at the other end of the bar and dance area until around 12 pm. I had been there on a number of occasions and I was dancing when I looked over and saw him. He was dark haired, with green eyes, a chiselled nose and extremely handsome. He was not difficult to spot as he was about 6 ft 5 inches tall and stood towering over everyone else. I caught his eye and he weaved his way through the dance floor towards me. I looked up at him and smiled and he asked if I would like a drink. Then he whispered in my ear "I really want your body" and snorted in a way that made me laugh. He used to wear 'Aramis' aftershave and years later I could always spot that smell from 20 yards.

We started dating albeit a very strange situation. He had a girlfriend who was a nurse and had been seeing her for some months. We used to see each other in a local pub/hotel and I would be with my friend Carol. She was about five foot two inches, and blonde with the most enormous breasts. We used to go out together every Friday and Saturday night and every time Dave would leave without his girlfriend and take me for a walk and start to kiss me. Even when he was with his girlfriend I would look over to him and give him that knowing look and off I would go to the ladies toilets. There he would follow me sneakily and steal a passionate kiss as I was returning.

On a few occasions he actually took me out on a date. It was usually in a pub with a bunch of his rugby player friends and I would return home around 3 am. One evening we were at the rugby club. He was drinking quite heavily and I was sitting on the bar stool in front of him, my legs spread so that he was standing between me. I was wearing black tights and a long black dress with ragged bottom and sleeves. I had made it myself especially for the evening. He was kissing me and touching my body all evening and he had the most amazing soft lips that sent shivers down my spine whenever he kissed me. At the end of the evening he walked me home across the fields, as my house was only about ten minutes walk away. As we reached the hedge he grabbed me and started to kiss my breasts. My nipples were hard and I started to feel shaky. He took me in his arms and removed my jacket and laid it on the floor. I lay down in front of him I feeling how cold the grass was through my clothing. He started to kiss me more passionately and then grabbed my breasts hard. He was rubbing my pussy through my panties and then lifted my dress up. I slid my underwear and pantyhose down and with my heels on I spread my legs. He started to unzip his trousers. I was feeling nervous and could not see much in the darkness. He did not touch my pussy but guided his cock into me. It slid in quite easily and I could feel his hardness inside me. I wanted him to kiss me an embrace me but he started to thrust for what seemed like about five minutes then suddenly he pulled out his cock and I felt a warm thrust of sperm on my leg. We did not speak and I hurried and dressed, pulling up my underwear and adjusting my dress. I felt disappointed and let down.

Was this what sex was all about five minutes of penetrations and no orgasm? After we walked home he kissed me goodnight on the doorstep and left. When I went to the bathroom to get changed I undressed and looked at my dress, which was black, and there was a large stain on the back of my dress. I started frantically trying to wash the stain away and the following morning

INTIMATE ENCOUNTERS

after I woke up the mark was still there. I remember thinking that sperm was difficult to remove and was worried in case my mother found my dress. We "dated" for about seven years during which time he must have had hundreds of other girlfriends.

I was living in London with a friend of mine called Clare having recently got back from my travels from living in a Kibbutz in Israel. Three of us had been renting a flat together in Kentish town and she has asked me if wanted to move in with her as she couldn't afford the rent. She was living in Dalston of all places. Dalston wasn't the trendy place up and coming place it is now it was a grotty dingy place in London that no one in their right mind wanted to live in. We stayed there for a couple of months sharing a basement flat with a roomful of snails that would that leave a trail on the carpet every morning and found a nice house share in Tottenham. There were about seven of us altogether and it was the first time in years I had moved all my things from my mother's house.

The weekend after I moved in we decided to go to Dingwells in Camden to see a band and it was late we couldn't afford a taxi and so I still had the keys from the flat in Kentish town as the guy that lived there worked abroad. We decided to stay out for the evening and sneak back to his flat and stay there for the night. Claire was a real air head she spent most of the day stoned making flower arrangements for the famous Kenny Everett show so it wasn't surprising that when we finally returned back to our house in Tottenham we were greeted by the smell of a burnt out building. While we had been out partying she had left her hair straighteners plugged in and the whole top floor had burnt down. The rest of the house guests weren't aware that we had actually gone out for the evening until we got back. Going into that room was heart wrenching. Seeing everything I had owned all gone up in a puff of smoke. All the dresses, the high heels, the jewellery, the records, the mementoes all burnt. I had played the classical guitar for years and there it was all charred and melted together. I never played the guitar again after the fire. It made me realize that material things really don't matter that much. It was only a room full of stuff but it was gone. I was reminded of the same thing later in my marriage when my husband who was very jealous was going through all my photographs. I had hundreds of pictures of me of all my travels, to Israel, Europe, Egypt, India and Nepal. Every picture he had found with me and another man on he destroyed. I remember crying and telling my mother and saying how could he do such a wicked thing and she said "its only pictures Rose. He can't take your memories away from you."

That week I became homeless Dave called me. I hadn't seen him for over a year as I had been away travelling. We always seemed to meet up every few months or years to catch up. He worked in a dead end job as an engineer whereas I was off gallivanting always wanting excitement and was off travelling somewhere new. He always said I inspired him and by that time he was now working as a successful teacher in Surrey. We talked for a while catching up and then he said "Well as you have no where to stay", he finally asked me to move in with him.

I thought about if for a few brief moments and suddenly everything fitted into place. In those seven years I had known him I travelled the world dated many men and deep down always had that dream that I would settle down and get married. I always had this dream I would live happily ever after like the fairy stories you read. My real name even means princess. How pathetic... how ridiculous. This man was just like my dad couldn't keep his cock in his trousers for one second and the irony was that on the odd few times we did actually sleep together in all those seven years it was always rubbish. I don't ever remember having an orgasm. I didn't even like him that much. We went away on holiday once for a week and he spent the whole week reading 'Lord of the Rings'. We didn't talk we didn't speak. The whole relationship was just based on looks and this "idea" of what I thought I wanted

All those years I had been in "love" with him and so desperate wanted to be married have the kids the whole works. Now he was finally asking me and all I could do was say "no thank you".

3 - THE HAPPY WANDERER

I left home in my teens, in hindsight I wanted to run away. From what? I am not sure, but I managed to manoeuvre myself halfway around the world with little else but a backpack and a few quid in my pocket. In my efforts to "find myself "I was in India when Gandhi got assassinated, I spent numerous nights drunk in a bomb shelter in Israel working as a volunteer, walked across the river Nile completely off my head on drugs in the hope that I might find myself and fell in love with a man who came from the other side of the world.

Being the middle child I have always been able to look after myself. I left school with 'O levels' having been to primary school and fast-tracked as a gifted child with an IQ that just failed to get me into Mensa. I remember my first week in senior school. I had done all this work when I was nine. I told the teacher and was told, "I am sorry but you have to do it all again". I guess that's why I wanted to travel. I didn't see the point doing a dead end job or going to university like my brothers doing a subject I had no interest in. I got bored easily so I would work for months on end taking 2 or 3 jobs at a time to earn enough money to go away for a few months. I lived all over London from the east end to the Kings Road moving from flat to flat in between travels. To me travelling was liberating, having a backpack and a bunch of mementoes from home was enough to make me feel secure.

INTIMATE ENCOUNTERS

I have had some of the most memorable experience whilst travelling which could fill a whole book on their own. I have walked the streets of Delhi on a curfew when there were no people around in the week that Gandhi was shot. I have sat next to lepers on a bus, during a lightning storm going around a hairpin bend on a half beaten bus up a mountain in Nepal. I have sat on a mountain top overlooking India where the Dalai Lama lives, I have lived on a houseboat in Kashmir, I have milked cows on a Kibbutz in Israel, been a volunteer making bomb shells have lived with the Palestinians in the Russian quarter, been arrested at the border for crossing 'No Mans Land', been locked up with two crazy Germans in some border town in Egypt while the border was closed and wasn't sure I could get out. Slept on a beach in Tell Aviv and woken up with the tide around my sleeping bag, stayed with a transvestite, lost a friend from 'Aids', been to wild parties in Goa when dance music wasn't even heard of. Sat and watched the moonlight alone when there was not a soul around on some quiet beach in India, travelled across Switzerland alone completely stoned and lost a day in my life and no idea where it went, been to China and worked in a hospital, seen and met some amazing people and sites, found myself, lost myself and not regretted a single moment of it.

I remember one incident in Nepal. I had been travelling for days, it was when you had to get long bus journeys, no two-hour flights, the temperature was a soaring 140 degrees. I had taken a minibus trip through the border from India through to Nepal. I was in the back of a dark minibus having changed buses a number of times. The travel companion I had left from England with I had met through 'Time Out' magazine. I remember our first meeting and thought he was gay and asked him. We had just been to Varanasi and they had a festival where they pour paint over the locals. I remember having pink hair for months after. Drugs were easily available in India and we had both drunk the local drink known as 'Bhang Lassi' a mixture of salt, yogurt milk shake mixed with grass. It gave you an incredible high. I had spent the week stoned visiting the 'Taj Mahal' daily looking at the wonderful colours how the marble changed during the different times during the day.

What an amazing place India was, so much wealth and so much poverty. Behind it was the remains of charred-out bodies that had been down the river from funeral pyres, the vultures pecking away at them. So Martin drunk the famous local drink and completely flipped out! I took him to the local homeopathic doctor who was somewhat confused as I tried to explain to him what he had drunk. He was totally off his head. It turns out he was gay and missed his boyfriend and he left me that week and flew back home to his boyfriend and had a complete breakdown. I saw him on my return and he admitted that he had had some issues and that probably going to India and getting high wasn't the answer. But then again I was still there, and I was feeling exhausted alone and stuck in some godforsaken border town.

I started to fall asleep and woke with a start with some Nepalese guys hands down my knickers trying to finger me while I was asleep on the bus. I screamed and ran to the front of the bus. We had arrived at the border and we were told it was closed and I had to stay overnight in a hotel. There was no one around who could speak proper English to listen to me so I somehow managed to book myself into some flea bitten hotel for the night. I put my rucksack next to the bed and went to check the door. I must have inadvertently not noticed what had happened as there were no lights in the room. When I slipped into bed there was a naked man laying on the bed. I don't remember much apart from screaming and kicking him out and reporting him to the border police who didn't even listen to me. As far as they were concerned I was a western woman travelling alone so I was easy game.

When I did finally reach Kathmandu I made my way to the centre of town. Tired and exhausted my Lonely Planet guide in hand for the nearest hotel and two hundred quid in my pocket to last the next four months. And then I don't remember anything. Apparently I had collapsed in the street. Some Nepalese people had picked me up and taken me to a local hotel. Luckily I hadn't been robbed, so someone was looking after me. Once I had recovered in Nepal I had a wonderful time. The people were friendly the scenery was amazing. At my lowest point I had had to phone home just after they had found me. Normally my mother answered but this time it was my dad. I wanted to tell him what happened, how I had nearly been raped, how I had just collapsed and how I desperately wanted to come home. Before I could even get past the Martins gone home bit he said "you know what Rose that's the one thing I like about you the adventurous spirit, your just like your dad a survivor, always brave always wanting to try something new" I didn't have the heart to tell him I wanted to come home so I kept quite. It wasn't until a year later and 3 stone lighter when I got back home; I realized I had contracted 'Giardia', parasites in the stomach from drinking dirty water. It took me years to get over my illness and I eventually went on to develop 'Chrohns' disease.

Did I mention briefly that I fell in love on my travels? The man in question was studying politics and when we first met it was love at first sight. It was a very hot day around 40 degrees. I was in Delhi at the time travelling which had a reputation for drug smugglers and had just been on the tail end of being planted with drugs and a free trip to Europe. In my naivety I had met a bunch of men from the Middle East who were over from Spain organizing their latest trip back. That included some poor unsuspecting European girl who would be the carrier, i.e. me.

I had been dating one of the men in question and in my naivety I was about to be duped before flying home. Sitting on the grass verge in the middle of the city in what was to be

INTIMATE ENCOUNTERS

known as the 'Tourist Camp' a friendly face came over to me and suggested that the people I had been mixing with were not exactly good company. He introduced himself as Bijan and explained that they were regular drug smugglers and wanted to use me as a courier. After unpacking my backpack numerous times and checking there was nothing suspicious I removed my belongings and placed it in a secure lock-up. I was due to fly home the next day so he offered me a coffee and we sat talking. I noticed a fair haired, dark tanned man of around twenty-four sitting away from me laughing and chatting to a couple of women. He was speaking English but with a very strong accent that I could not fathom. I could not keep my eyes off him and asked Bijan if he knew the man and said jokingly he is gorgeous and assumed that he was not Middle Eastern. Bijan replied that he was and that he was also his friend and introduced us.

His name was Alex and we talked and laughed for what seemed like hours and I had the feeling I had known him forever. In the evening we were alone and after we made love for the first time I remember saying to him that when we were old and grey I would be looking after him. I had to fly back and returned to the UK a couple of days later. On my return to the UK I managed to get myself a job with a temping agency and a couple of nights a week as a barmaid plus a weekend job as a controller for a local cab firm. Three months later and £1000 in the bank I was back on the plane to see Alex. We would spend three months together on a beach living simply in a beach hut, eating local prawn salads, enjoying the sun, making love, getting high and partying at night.

He had the most insatiable sex drive. We would often make love 4-5 times a day.

When I returned home for the second time I was desperate to see him again and he promised me as soon as his studies were over he would fly over. I wrote to him every couple of days but as soon as I realized I wasn't going to get any reply after a few months I started to try and rebuild my life. I was living in a hostel in the centre of London and decided it was time to move on and find myself a flat. I had been there for over a year since my return and was enthusiastic about the future. As I was leaving the hostel that day the receptionist called me and said he had a letter for me. I hurriedly grabbed the letter and looked at the scribbled handwriting on the envelope. As I opened it my heart fell. It was a letter from Alex; he had been in the country for a couple of months and wanted to meet up. I decided to call him and he explained that he was sorry for not contacting me before but had had some problems with his family and decided to come here and see me. Could not understand why he had taken six months to contact me but nonetheless we started up where we had left off.

It was about six months into the relationship when I was waiting at a bus stop and saw a blonde woman standing there and I recognized her instantly. We had met previously on our travels in India and she had been living with Alex's

INTIMATE ENCOUNTERS

friend for a couple of months in San Francisco. We started to chat and it transpired that during the time I was with him, no sooner had I jumped on the plane to return home, he was greeting another woman from the UK and spent a couple of months with her. Also the reason he had not contacted me for so long was because he had been living with her and planned to marry. I was completely devastated that he could have cheated on me so I ended the relationship shortly after.

Rose Budworth Levine

4 - MY LOST YEARS

A few months went by and I was back on the dating scene. I had been seeing an American oil tycoon who was married. I like it that way as there was no emotional attachment and we used to spend nights making love on his trips over to the UK. It was around that time that I bumped into Alex and we ended up making love at the end of a very emotional reunion. I told him it was a mistake and that I didn't want to see him again. A few weeks later I was starting to feel unwell so I went to see my doctor who informed me that I was pregnant, I was twenty-two and I had no idea whether the father was the adulterous American or Alex. I was so hurt by what he had done to me the last thing I wanted to do was have his child so I promptly booked myself in for an abortion. My father took me in and collected me that evening. I cried a little and thought no more of it and decided as soon as I felt better to go away on holiday for a week.

I managed to find a last minute booking to Tunisia and spent the week reading books and lazing on the beach. I met a man who was about forty-five. He was married and worked at Heathrow as a policeman and we made love a few times before I returned home. I made a promise to myself never to go out with a foreigner again.

My father collected me from the airport and took me back to my flat. I asked him to stop on the way for some milk and tea because I knew the flat was empty and wandered around the shop

INTIMATE ENCOUNTERS

aimlessly. Two men were standing there chatting in a language I knew quite well from my time with Alex. I wandered up to them and started to talk and they asked me which part of the country I was from. I explained I was not Middle Eastern but English and they passed me their telephone number and said if you fancy a drink call us.

A week or so passed by and I called and we arranged to meet up. They were both good fun and I was flattered by their attention. I couldn't decide which one I wanted to date so I plumped for the short 'Danny DeVito look-alike' that made me laugh. It was early one night in February and we had arranged for all three of us to meet up for a drink. We were sitting chatting in the pub when 'Danny' said they had a friend they were meeting and would I like to go to a party with them all. As I looked across the room, this gorgeous dark stranger walked in. I could not help but catch my breath when I saw him. He smiled at me and walked over towards us. After the customary kiss on each cheek to introduce himself he said hello and sat next to me. His name was Mahmoud and I realized his English was not good. We sat for a while, then the others started to talk in their own language and we all went and followed him out, and drove to the party. The party was hosted by his ex-girlfriend, a forty something woman with long dark hair. Most of the people there were Middle Eastern. I sat next to him all evening trying hard to converse with him and using lots of body language and gestures to make myself understood.

Rose Budworth Levine

The first night I had sex with Mahmoud was interesting to say the least although it didn't set a president for the rest of what was going to become a very long marriage. The 'Danny DeVito look-alike' I had been seeing was off working in Scotland and had been there for a week or so. I remember him telling me to behave myself and keep my legs crossed while I was away which made me laugh. I couldn't stop thinking about Mahmoud and found a crumpled bit of paper in the bottom of my handbag. I even recall calling my mother and telling her how I had met this wonderful man and her asking for his name. She said "mmmm that sounds very middle eastern" I laughed and said it was. She asked how long I had been seeing him and I said I hadn't been out with him yet, but I would soon. I guess sometimes you just know when things are meant to happen. So I called up his friend Ali and asked if Mahmoud was in. Arrived at his door and Ali was dressed to go out. He left us alone, one large bottle of vodka Smirnoff in the middle of the coffee table. Two total strangers, albeit we had met briefly the week before at a party that could hardly converse and half a bottle later we had ripped each others clothes off and were fucking each others brains out on a pile of washing on his friend Ali's bed.

It was in the early days that I had met Ali, who was Mahmoud's closest friend. He wasn't the happiest of people and despite numerous attempts on both Mahmoud's and my part including one visit to his flat where we found him slumped over the toilet injecting himself in his balls because all his other veins had collapsed sadly he succumbed to a life of heroin and later died of aids.

I met many friends through my travels who dabbled with drugs. I even dabbled with them myself. I thought I will try everything once. Those drugs I tried that were too enticing, like cocaine, I tried only a couple of times and then never took them again. I guess I needed that control just to see what it was like. We all find ourselves addicted to something in our lives, be it cigarettes destructive relationships, sex, I guess drugs just weren't for me.

I spent most of my teenage life on drugs of some sort, those of the prescription kind. I had always been big for my age. Both big from a size point of view and big from a weight point of view well at least that's what the charts said. My father had a thing about me being overweight so I used to go to the doctor and was put on "sponsored slims" to encourage me to lose weight. My dad would always say I will give you a pound for every pound you lose. I don't know why he was so obsessed with me being overweight, maybe because he had been an overweight child himself, who knows. Looking back I was about a size 14 which for someone who is over 5' 8" is quite average but never the less the doctor seemed to think that 'Dospan' and 'Apisate' seemed like good pills to put me on. So I spent much of my teenage years popping slimming pills and water retention tablets that would help lose weight and I could piss for England. Sure I lost weight but I piled it on when I came off of them. I found out later that both 'Dospan' and 'Apisate' are now banned drugs and maybe that was part of what started my downward spiral of depression and suicidal thoughts. The first most prominent one aged around 17.

I started my periods at age 11, although was warned that I may start as early as nine. I remember having "tummy ache" and my first period was at secondary school. It was in my "RE" lesson. I was later to find I had 'Endometriosis' and 'Fibroids' but at the time wasn't quite sure what was happening when even with all the preparation from my mother and the doctors I found myself, tampax inserted, pads inside my underwear a pairs of tights and another pair of knickers over the top the blood flooding through my skirt and the boys laughing because there was a nice red patch on the back of my skirt. I had to go to the ladies room and took off all my underwear and skirt and washed it and put it on the old Victorian style radiator to try and dry it off. Obviously I was late for class and was greeted by the stupid "RE teacher" saying "and where do you think you have been Miss Budworth-Levine?" and all the boys sniggering because they just knew.

I was put on the pill at twelve to try and control my periods which didn't help and spent years in and out of hospital having it all sucked out, or more technically speaking having a "D and C" to try and fix me up until I was eventually fobbed off and told the only way I could fix it was to have babies but since there was almost no chance of that having had 4 or 5 miscarriages during my marriage I guess I was gob smacked when I finally did become pregnant. I had been due to go into hospital the following week for yet another "D and C" when I didn't feel right. I did a couple of pregnancy tests which both came out negative then finally called the doctor who did a blood test which showed I was pregnant. I even bled during that. I went to the doctor and was told the baby had died and to go and home and wait for it to come out. So I did. I was working for an American Stock Brokers at the time and lost my job in the process due to having so much time off work. When I went back to hospital to check that it was all gone there was a heartbeat. No miscarriage but a healthy baby growing inside me who was to become my daughter Emma.

Mahmoud always wanted a daughter, it was all he ever dreamed about which was strange because most men from the Middle East always just want a son. He had arrived in England just out of a civil war and we had been together more than five years. I guess I married him because he made me feel safe, He was quite different from Alex, he wasn't like my father and there was just me and him, but in some ways especially when I look back he was very controlling. I had a great job working in the city, I was always the "bread winner", I think he was quite liberal and tolerate, but the chink in his amour would show when I would mention something innocent, like I had gone to lunch with my boss, or been out with friends. Gradually during the first five years of marriage I dropped all my friends one-by-one. I didn't even realize I was doing it at first. I had never met any of his family apart from his sister who worked for an airline and used to pop over every so often. I knew he came from a very large family of ten brothers and sisters, a matriarchal mother and father who had left them all when they were small. Two of his brothers were living in another country and desperate to come to England as refugees so I helped Mahmoud to bring both of them over. The authorities were being very difficult and the political situation was very tense. I guess because I had a decent job it probably helped so I contacted a solicitor and paid for them to help them into the country. I was three months pregnant with my daughter when they finally arrived. We had moved from a small flat in east London to a huge big house that we could hardly afford in order to accommodate the new family that was arriving. Little did I know how big a family we were about to accommodate.

It was with some trepidation and shock when I found that not only were his two brothers now living with me but his sister and her two children and his mother were soon to arrive within the same month. Mahmoud's sister had decided to leave her husband for a better life in the UK and bring along her mother. Not once did Mahmoud ask me was if it was OK for them to move in.

My youngest brother John had been staying with me for a while and had just returned back home to my mum as he couldn't cope with the high life living in London and had become hooked on dope and was taking coke and ecstasy.

INTIMATE ENCOUNTERS

Often he would call in a pretty sorry state not knowing where he was or even what day it was working for a busy advertising agency in the city. I worked for a stockbrokers and I had fallen pregnant shortly after when Mahmoud's brothers had arrived. His sister arrived about a month later with her two kids and then there was the mother-in-law. If I could describe the mother-in-law from hell it had to be Mahmoud's mother. She was some matriarchal type woman who was power-driven, having bought up the children on her own. I realized just how manipulative she was when I made a comment to my sister-in-law one day, on how great my mother in laws figure was on having had ten children but commenting on the big scar across the middle of her tummy. She told me that one of the sons had misbehaved so the mother had swallowed a packet of sewing needles and had to have her stomach cut open. On another occasion she has poured petrol over herself because one of the boys had not done what she asked of them. Mary Mahmoud's sister, had made a promise to look after her mother, after begging her not to kill herself, and hence the reason the family were so afraid of their mother. They all openly hated her but deep down still loved her because she was their mother. Then there was me, heavily pregnant, hormones all over the place, I had just lost my job and I had the whole crazy bunch of them living with me in my house.

Six months ago it had been just me and Mahmoud looking forward to a future together with our new baby and now we had this whole family of our own and I didn't even ask for them to be there. Mahmoud was starting to act very strange almost reverting back to his old ways. I had to start acting differently making sure I behaved properly in front of his mother. They would complain about the fact that I had cats, and say they were dirty, they would accuse me of being a terrible housewife and say my house was dirty and filthy. They wouldn't eat the food I cooked them and ate in separate rooms. They talked amongst themselves in their own language and made me feel like I wasn't even there.

Our debts were spiralling out of control the mortgage rate was about 14.5 percent. I had always been the breadwinner paying for Mahmoud and I to go on nice holidays and enjoy ourselves. I didn't have a nice cushy mortgage subsidy to go with my job anymore, as I was now redundant. Mahmoud had lost his job too and was self-employed doing whatever he could to makes ends meet. The food bills had increased and the phone bill was enormous. Then he wanted another member of the family to come with his wife and three children. It was at that point when I had finally had my baby, I think she was about 3 months old when I decided to speak to one of the brothers. I told him the pressure on Mahmoud was too much and he was going to have a breakdown not to mention me. He was already on anti-depressants and under a lot of stress to pay all the bills. His mother watched and listening in her half understanding of English. Mehdi seemed to be sympathetic he said he would speak with the family and left. I was left alone in the house with the baby and his mother. She started to talk to me in half English half Persian saying how I was selfish and how all I cared about was money. She said "What about the money you spend on your cigarettes and your cats. God, how my mother-in-law hated those cats. Our food bills were enormous and our phone bills all to the Middle East. I am a very placid person and I picked up the baby and tried to explain myself but it just got worse, she just kept on and on. Eventually she was starting to go, crazy spitting on the floor and drawing crosses and saying, "he is my son, you are nothing, you are not part of the family, and he is my baby." She was of course referring to her son, my husband. At that point I told her to get out of my house. She replied "You get out". I wanted to slap her but instead I called Mahmoud. He never took my side, said she was an old lady that I should respect and even if she had hit me I should accept it.

I wasn't having that. I stayed there for another 9 months until one day Mahmoud came home from work and I was gone. I had packed up everything and my father came and collected all my things. He didn't even call me for two weeks he said later "I knew you were at your mother's." We reconciled, god knows why and I went back for another couple of years. There was always the promise of things changing but I spent the rest of my marriage running a business for him that his family would end up taking over and using us as a bank.

When we had our second child I was working by the time he was six months old running the shop again. The child minder wasn't available that week and Mahmoud was on holiday and we always holidaying apart. He was always off with his friends with some excuse saying he was on business. It was Turkey this time buying up some land with money I never saw. I had the baby in the pushchair running the shop with his youngest brother and we had a huge row. He said his family think I am just using Mahmoud for money and that I have a private bank account tucked away, as he was always telling them that there was never any money to give them. All of them were fucked up by their own manipulative mother, playing one-off against the other. Mahmoud wasn't a mean person but he just never put me or the kids first. We had his friend called Fardi living with us for a couple of years while my daughter was still little. She hated him so much. He was a drug addict although he never took drugs while he was in our house he was an opium smoker. He was down on his luck lost, his job as a lorry driver through a back injury, and during the time that he stayed with us Mahmoud would always bung him a tenner whenever he was skint. It was two years later and we had moved into an ex-council property in west London. It was a Four-bedroom house with the opportunity to purchase at a price of £83,000. Having lost the home we lived in previously being repossessed it seemed like an ideal opportunity for us to get back everything we had lost. Things were looking up. We had just cleared off all our debts and needed money to pay the deposit and solicitors fees. So when Fardi came with £1,500 saying to Mahmoud this is the money I owe you for all the time you have given me money for the last two years I was delighted. See, that's how Mahmoud was easy as giving stuff away he didn't have. That week I asked Mahmoud for the money for the solicitor and he said "its gone" I asked him "where, where's it gone?" He had used the money to pay for his brothers wedding. As soon as his mother had found out about the money she had booked a hotel up near Holland Park to impress everyone. Ironic really when our own wedding was me and him, and my family, and not a single present in site from any of them. I remember talking to my sister in law in question who got married that day saying "are you sure you want to marry into this family". She was Turkish and obviously they loved her because she wasn't English like me. She had suffered the marriage for 7 years. Now she is 4 stone overweight, has no self-esteem and I just look in the mirror and see her as being like myself.

With the business sold I decided I would tell him I would go back and work in the city. I used to work as a consultant teaching windows and ran a computer network doing support for a large city stockbroker. I had been out for over seven years. He said, "You will never be able to stick it". He was right after a month of temping I hated the city and it wasn't until I went back to work that I realized what I had left in the first place. It was a retrace so I decided to take a huge brave decision and start retraining as an alternative therapist. It was a two year full-time course. My son Francis was 9 months old and it would mean me going back to school after twenty years. I managed to get a grant and had a touch interview from the head teacher as I was very ill at the time and they didn't see how I would be able to manage a full-time course with two kids. I started the course and was amazed that I had forgotten who I was all the time I had been married. I had lost all my friends and started to make new ones. My confidence increased and my husband started seeing a different me. I had been there for a few months working hard and getting straight A's in my assignments. Juggling the children and making sure I didn't rock the boat at home as I was looking forward to doing something worthwhile, a job I might actually enjoy and get paid for. I made plans to set up a business from home when we finished and buying our house was the perfect answer.

One month later the house we wanted was bought with money borrowed from my father as he knew I a hard time over the past few years living from door-to-door in council flats and losing everything. I felt positive; we even talked about moving to America, being near my brother Sean and starting afresh without his family hanging round his neck to ponse off him. He left me that week. I moved to my mothers the next month, as there was no money to pay for the mortgage I had to let the house out. I lived the next year in two rooms and drove 600 miles a week to finish my course.

For all his generosity to his family I walked away from the house and left him with half of everything, never fought him in court, He came out of the marriage with £100,000 cash and managed to spend most of in the a couple of years. He came back a few years later when he was down on his luck and stupidly I got persuaded into letting him buy a house I should have had the guts to buy myself. More than £100,000 profit later and a portfolio of properties left him quite wealthy. Me, well I was such a mug, the maintenance payments came few and far between, I hadn't gone to court so my debts started to spiral.

My sex life with my husband left a lot to be desired to say the least. A handsome fit man I fancied right up until well after my divorce from him. I always had to initiate any sexual contact. His usual excuse was he was tired or had things on his mind. For many years I thought he was having an affair, I even thought he was gay at one point as he was always happy in the company of his male friends.

He came from a strict Muslim background and although he had given up the faith many years ago I felt sure he had many hang-ups about his sexuality. His idea of foreplay was to put a finger inside me to check I was wet then he would have sex with me for maybe ten minutes or so until he prematurely ejaculated. His excuse for coming so quickly was that he was so excited and fancied me so much he couldn't control himself. If that was the case then why did he hardly sleep with me? Apart from the beginning we used to make love about once a month. If I tried to instigate love making, on the rare occasion more than once a week he would remind me that it wasn't good to have sex too much and that he would lose his hair. Sometimes it made me laugh and sometimes I just thought it was his way of controlling me because he knew I had a huge appetite for sex and would have been happy to have sex every night of the week. He always said I never once said no to him throughout our marriage.

It was always spur of the moment quickies when I could manage to persuade him. He never looked at porn and said it was disgusting. God forbid that I would ever masturbate although towards the end of the marriage I did start to but I always felt disgusting and guilty. The first thing I did when I was divorced was go and buy myself a vibrator. It was amazing that such a small thing could make me come so quickly and I named them my plastic boyfriends.

We never did foreplay apart from me giving him lots of oral sex then he would use that excuse too and say I was so wonderful he couldn't help but come. As far as giving me pleasure he would never dream of "going down there" as he called it. That made me feel dirty and I had a real hang-up about my sexuality for many years. Sometimes we would discuss it or rather I would try and broach the subject but I always ended up wishing I had never started the conversation. The intimacy disappears after the first few years and we never kissed because he had a sinus problem and he said that he couldn't breath properly. It was always a kiss and a hug. Eventually we ended up sleeping in separate beds for the last 5 or so years of our marriage. He was on one of the sofas and I was upstairs on my own trying to hold back the tears. How many tears I cried after we made love feeling that total disappointment and knowing that five minutes of passion would be over and he would leave my bed and go sleep in another room. He always said it was because he was a light sleeper and I disturbed his talking in my sleep which kept him awake. No wonder I was to explore my sexuality to the full when I was single although I was to have one more marriage before I was brave enough to do it.

5 - SOULMATES NEED NOT APPLY

"I will divorce you with the same passion I did when I first met you". These were the last words I said to my second husband Alex. I guess those words will resonate and torment for the rest of his miserable life.

Some of us have a habit of going back into our past when things are down it makes us feel secure. After I had left Mahmoud with two kids in tow and no maintenance I finished my course then ended up in hospital with Chrohns disease. It was probably the stress of the break-up. I had been told by the doctors I had chronic Chrohns and that I would be ill for the rest of my life. But I am a firm believer in mind-over-matter and spent weeks visualizing, I have two friends who have the disease and the ultimate end is to end up with cancer or have a colostomy bag. I kept telling myself there is no way I am going to end up with a bag and kept willing it away. Two months later I told the specialist I was no longer taking the tablets and that the Chrohns had gone. He said "Rose you cant just get rid of it like that" So I suggested he did a scan. A couple of weeks later the results were back and he said "Well I don't know what you have done Rose but there is no sign of any Chrohns any more". To this day I have never had another proper attack.

Life has a way of bringing things into our life when we least expect it and I had bumped into a friend from India and it was my brother Sean's second wedding. I was going to see him when he suggested I go visit an old mutual friend who was living there. His name was Patrick and he was living in San Francisco. I met him briefly with his new wife and children and he explained that my old boyfriend Alex who I had fallen in love with many years ago in India was now living in Canada.

It goes without saying that I started talking to him on the phone, after 17 years and six months later I was in Canada visiting him. Five months after that I was there with my two children and we got married mainly because I thought it would be easier to sort out the paperwork. People never really change; they get older and hopefully wiser. He had been living there, wasting his life doing nothing. He even had the same old clothes he had been wearing in London, the double-breasted designer suits he had worn to woo all those many women he had bedded before. He hadn't managed to find a proper job in Canada even though he was educated and spoke nearly seven languages so I helped him redo his CV, chucked out all his clothes and went out with my daughter on a shopping spree Came back 150 dollars later with a whole range of stylist outfits for him to go for interview. Motivated and fired up he got himself a job the next week as a manager in a shop. We talked about how things had been in the past and how with a strong woman like me would have made his life completely different,

I thought in my own twisted way I was his saviour, that everything that had gone in the past could be put right. He seemed sorry he had cheated on me. He seemed sorry that all those years had been spent wasting his life. He was upset that he had never married and explained that the reason he had never wanted to be my wife before was because I had been told I couldn't have children. Now he saw me with two gorgeous intelligent children, he saw how unhappy my marriage had been, he wanted to make amends. It was a like a true fairy tale ending.

But as everyone knows fairy tales are just bollocks and Princes don't grow up and marry Princes, and chances are I had married a frog. It was the most freezing cold winter in Canada's history for 40 years. We had no car and I had to take the bus with the kids to the equivalent of Kwik Save to buy the weekly shopping. The paperwork he had promised to sort out hadn't been done. Meanwhile my ex-husband found out who I had married and was accusing me of cheating on him throughout our marriage and threatened me and the children and said he would get us arrested. We were rapidly running out of money and I realized I would have to come back home. Unfortunately Alex had a secret habit, which soon became obvious. He was an opium user and I found out years later he had been using it most of his adult life. Opium is a great drug; I have tried it once or twice. It takes away all your pain and makes you talk complete shit. Makes you think you can do anything and it might even make other people believe it too because you don't even look like your stoned most of the time. It turns you into a complete bullshitter and procrastinator of the highest order. I found out he was smoking after we had married and told him I never wanted him smoking again with my children in the house. His behaviour started to be a bit erratic from then on. I went back to England and he was supposed to sort out his paperwork to come and live here with the children and me. I hadn't finalized my divorce money. I had a lot of debts to pay off. He was talking the talk but I couldn't see whether he was doing the talk as I was too busy when I got back home finding a job and sorting everything out for when he came back over to the UK.

The authorities would not give him a visa until we could prove our finance which had been in a bit of a state, as I had sold everything up and moved over there and not worked for 4 months and then had to ship it al back again. It was seven months and I finally sorted out my finances and had secretly arranged to buy a house, pay off my debts and call and surprise him. I didn't want him to know what I had been doing; I just wanted him to work hard at kicking the drugs and coming over. I called him at work and it was busy so I decided to call home and leave a message for him to call. A woman answered the phone; he was obviously having an affair. When I confronted him he said she was probably someone trying to rob him and that they had picked up the phone! And then he tried to turn it around and accuse me of having an affair. I just laughed and said look you know. You are talking to someone that has a father that has cheated on my mum so many times. I had learnt well from my fathers lying and I knew every trick in the book.

I filed for divorce the next week. I never heard from him for two years in fact they didn't even find him to give him the divorce papers. I got out of the blue one day from a lawyer saying he was trying to sue me for 50,000 dollars. The furniture I had left there for him to sell and the rent he had not paid had been put on his credit cards. He hadn't paid anything in four years just the minimum payments. When she called and I explained what had happened and how I had come back to England with £20,000 worth of debt had cleared it all off and now I was settled I told her I would get one penny over my dead body.

One year on from my break up with Alex and I thought I was ready to have a relationship again. Only this time I decided it would be different. I would choose men completely different from my ex husbands and I would also ensure that I never got involved with anyone emotional. I had been using the Internet for sometime mostly just playing really, when I remembered an incident that had happened with Alex in Canada. It was late at night and he was to work at 6 am. I am a bit of a night owl and could not sleep and had decided to download some music from a site. There was a music chatroom attached to the site and I thought it would be interesting to go in, I think I picked alternative 80s pop. I had never used a chat room before and I was surprised to find lots of private message popping up saying a/s/l. I had not idea what they were talking about so responded by saying no. Then I decided to browse on another site and look up Chat room terminology. It was then that I realized that asl mean age sex location. I was so embarrassed having used computers for nearly 20 years that I had no idea what it meant I quickly logged off the pc. As I was closing down I could hear Alex walking down the corridor. He asked me what I had been doing and I explained that I was downloading music and had accidentally gone into a chatroom. Then a barrage of abuse followed with him accusing me of having cybersex on the net. I was so angry that he would accuse me of something like that but it was then that I remembered some of the things he had dropped into the conversation when we first started chatting on the net. We had a huge row and I realized then that he had been chatting to underage girls on the net and that was why he knew so much about chat rooms. It was his guilt that led him to accuse me as I believe as he could not be trusted he must have thought that the rest of the world was like him.

I was disgusted and we never spoke for a week after that incident. So when I was back in England, my relationship over, I started to think about all the things I had been accused of and wondered what all this "cybersex" was all about. I found a chat room called Flirt, which was an animated version of a normal chat room. I found it very amusing as the people in the room used symbolic images as representations of themselves. For example one of the women would use pictures of Cristina Aguilera when in fact in real life she was a brunette, married with 3 children and weighed about 20 stone. I used to go into the chat room every day and started talking to an Israeli man who was about 23 years old and unhappily married.

We had lots of things in common, the same taste in music and I felt at ease chatting too him. Neither of us had any idea what each other looked like but the conversations soon had a sexual connotation and was my first experience of "cybersex". What surprised me was that this was a man I knew nothing about, who was on the other side of the world, who made me feel flattered by his attention and that I through words alone he could make me orgasm.

On a couple of occasions we would be in the middle of conversation and he would say that he had come and then log off the computer immediately. The following day he would be embarrassed and say that he had heard his wife coming in and that she had nearly caught him masturbating. A few weeks followed and the guilt set in and I never saw him online again. His email address disappeared and he was gone.

After my brief experimentation with "cybersex" I decided it was not for me and that to have the sexual attention I craved I would need to actually meet someone. I added myself to a number of dating sites and got a number of emails from desperate men wanting relationships because their previous partner had been unfaithful or they had come to a point in their life when they perhaps wanted to settle down. It was then that I stumbled on a site that had three sections. One was dating; the second relationships and the third entitled "Intimate Encounters". I browsed the site to get a feel for what people were looking for and decided to place and advertisement. At first I had no photograph and my login name was "Shy "one which I found highly amusing as I am not in the least bit shy. I was very clear about what I wanted emphasizing that I was looking for someone that would be willing to take time and please me sexually with lots of foreplay. I also mentioned that although I was not looking for Mr Right if something developed I would be happy to progress onto a relationship. I convinced myself that after 15 years of sex with little or no foreplay now was not the time to enjoy myself. My advert read like this:

'PLEASE READ MY PROFILE FIRST AND NOT JUST LOOK AT MY PICS
SOULMATES NEED NOT APPLY'

"I guess from the sarcastic few I should be on dateline but then I am on here because I am an adult and I can! I am looking for a man that knows how to please a woman   A man that doesn't think his idea of foreplay is two fingers and a fuck. I guess I am looking for a man that likes to eat me real slow!

If I do ever find a man to have a relationship I will have gotten the important bit out of the way first.   I am however looking for a long term relationship.

For anyone that does venture past this bit I they will find an adventurous, intelligent, sexy 40 year old with a fuller figure who is also very open-minded when it comes the subjects of the adult kind.

On the other hand, I am also easy going, caring, considerate and will give my undivided attention to the right man.

Looking to meet a genuine unattached, intelligent attractive man for a 1 on 1 relationship and then who knows maybe move onto something more adventurous.

So if you are looking for a quickie, cybersex, you are married, have a girlfriend, or married to your job DO NOT REPLY. I have heard it all before. I am a real person with real feelings too.

If you cant be bother to send a decent picture and a thoughtful reply then I wont reply either. I am not that impressed by private part shots."

It was a complete contradiction. What I wanted was non consensual adult fun but at the reality was that deep down I wanted a loving committed relationship but I had been so disappointed with my choices and failed marriages I couldn't bear falling in love again.

A couple of days later I logged into the PC to check if I had an emails and was surprised to find more than 100 emails in my inbox and an open ended chat room with more than 70 people wanting to talk to me. Some of the emails I received said nice arse wouldn't mind getting my tongue round that. Others didn't bother even reading the profile as most of them were married and had girlfriends. Some opening lines were I love to eat real slow. Some of the replies were just plain revolting.   Or I would get a load of emails with pictures of guys cocks attached to the email. No face just a cock as if that was saying something profound.   I have never particularly liked the way English men communicated with women and it amused me to read some of the chat up lines they used.   I guess I was guilty of encouraging crude comments as on the particular site just from my profile.   Everyone had an opening line.   Some would use sentences like "sensual, erotic man looking for fun" "grab your coat, you have pulled" ETC ETC.

Then having waded through the responses that would fall into my inbox daily I stumbled and a very nice email from a 23-year-old man.   It was not crude or disgusting like some of the other emails I had been receiving and he went on to explain that he would love to find a woman that was older than himself and enjoyed ladies with a larger than average figure which delighted me. We spoke on the phone and he was quite nervous but we arranged to meet the following week. I was under no misconception; I had it in my mind that if there was some chemistry I would be willing to have sex with this 23 year old stranger I had found on the net. I drove to where he lived about 30 minutes away since he had no car and was a student. I saw him walking down the street, he was about 5 10, attractive, dark hair and eyes with a muscular build. He walked towards the car and I wound down the window. He leaned inside the car and kissed me passionately. A rush of adrenaline and excitement went through my body as I drove in silence, him at my side back to my house.

We chatted nervously for an hour or so and then started to kiss me and said please lay on the floor. I knew that he wanted to undress me and he started to kiss my breasts and move his hands and tongue all over my body. He started to remove my trousers and as I lay there feeling excited and helpless he started to work his way down my stomach with his tongue. He parted my legs and said I want to lick you. My heart was racing, I was so nervous, all I could think of was the thoughts I previously had from being married about oral sex, and how maybe there was something wrong with me, and that if he was to taste me it would disgust him. A million thoughts raced through my head, but I wanted him so badly. His head was now between my legs and the anticipation was too much for me I wanted to move away but he wrapped his hands underneath my thighs and brought my pussy towards him. As he started to lick and tease my lips and clitoris the sensation was so intense I came within minutes. I thought he was going to stop but he continued for minutes after minutes. He started to devour me and made me orgasm in a way I had never had before. He would kiss my thighs and then started all over again. I could feel the wetness of my orgasm trickling down my leg and he would start eagerly to lick me again. I felt like I was in heaven and at one point I came so much I wanted to cry. His tongue was expert like a crescendo of waves upon my eager pussy. I felt like years of sexual tension had been released.

Many orgasms later and for what seemed like an eternity, but turned out to be around 90 minutes, he finally released my pussy with his mouth and looked up at me between my legs. He said that I had the most wonderful tasting pussy he had ever licked and it was then that I burst into tears. He looked at me and asked why I was crying. I explained that I had been in an unhappy relationship for a long time and that my partner had never wanted or even tried to have oral sex with me. I explained how I had thought there was something wrong with me. He was wonderful he explained that he really enjoyed pleasuring a woman and that he had met a few women in the past that he had given oral sex to but that none was as responsive and sweet tasting and that there was nothing he would rather do than pleasure me. We then proceeded to make love to each other for the best part of the day. And after I drove him back home I returned home feeling exhilarated but a little empty because his body was not there to wake up next to.

We continued to see each other for a couple of months and he would call me often and chat on the Internet between meetings. I decided after a couple of months to finish the relationship as there was never going to be any way we would end up being together. As a person he was not confident but as a lover he was extremely giving. I felt that what we had during those months was that we were seeing each other and learning a lot about ourselves. I had learnt about my insecurities about being older and not having the perfect body, He had learnt much from me about sex and lack of confidence.

Many months later when I was chatting again to him on the internet he told me that I had changed his life. He explained that I had made him feel good about himself and given him the confidence to go and have relationships with other women. He had also gotten more confident with his relationships with his parents who had suffocated him over many years and he was ready to start a new life.

What transpired after that encounter was a string of encounters over the internet that were to change the way I viewed men forever, at least that was what I thought. Throughout my life men have always wanted me for sex and those that haven't I married them. Quite a contrast to the way most people see relationships. I always wanted a special bond with someone, someone I could be a friend with but at the same time be their lover. I was growing in confidence with regards to being by myself and not having that ache there that needed to be filled by having someone live with me.

Because I always wanted that special relationship and then when I had it seemed so disappointing or I felt like I was doing it all wrong. I thought the only way to resolve it was to work my way through my emotions and detach myself from the emotional bond that came with sexual contact and intimate relationships. I wanted to explore, and by doing this it took me on a soul-searching journey that would awaken the innermost feelings I had as a woman.

I started by going on a dating site. Not the normal dating site you would imagine it was an adult dating site. After the advert I had previously placed going under the name of "Shyone", which seemed ironic really as I was never shy. I would check my inbox daily to see if there were any possible suitors. I had been chatting via email to a man called Steve who said he was into extreme snowboarding and paragliding. He sounded excited and pretty well rounded not the normal type on that site that was just of for sex so we had arrange to meet in a couple of weeks.

During the time I was corresponding with him I had been watching the television it was the Para-Olympics. A very handsome looking man appeared from nowhere and I remember thinking how did he get to where he was. I had chatted to Steve for sometime when he revealed that he had some difficulty walking and that he would need access for his chair. It seemed strange when he had mentioned that he did snowboarding earlier. I never really thought anything of it until the day he came to see me in his wheelchair. I was shocked more than anything so we chatted and we had a coffee. We were busy discussing life in general and he mentioned that he had been a motorcyclist who had taken one too many risks. After his accident he became paralysed from the waist down and was unable to have any kind of sexual relationship. He had spent the last few years doing dangerous sports despite his disability and he was a participant in the Olympic games. That's when I realized who he was. The same man I had seen on the television a few weeks earlier.

We sat on the sofa and chatted a while. Interestingly enough he had a pierced tongue because he said the only way he could pleasure a woman was through oral sex. I had the overwhelming urge to kiss him and although he was implying that he gained pleasure from pleasing a woman I just wanted to give him some pleasure. I sat on his lap and started to kiss him on the lips. Just then I felt this dampness. He looked embarrassed and explained that he was totally incontinent and that whilst I had maneuvered myself onto his lap I had inadvertently released the contents of his urinal bag onto my sofa.

Poor guy, how sorry I felt for him. We didn't see each again after that but we continued for some time to speak to each other on the internet and I found out later he had moved to Canada to start a new life as a disabled coach.

I continued with the whole internet chat with numerous different men. Most of whom I never met, most of whom were married, and most of who just wanted some cyber fantasy to take them away from there illus ional lives. I had profiles on a number of different sites with a number of different disguises.

INTIMATE ENCOUNTERS

I wanted to find out how men thought what made them tick. I wanted to discover what stirred them and what they really thought about women. Most of the men I chatted to via email and instant messenger were either disillusioned divorcees who wanted no strings fun or married men that were getting their kicks from chatting on the internet. I have always been very faithful in any relationship and I found it very hard to understand why these men would want to have intimate chats about their wildest fantasies with a woman they had never met. The reality through talking to various people was that most of the women who had profiles on dating sites, swinging sites were in fact men.

I remember having a wonderful chat on messenger one night with this "woman" who told me how much she loved being bisexual and wanted to meet me. Only to realize that at some point during our conversations she was actually a man.

I was about to go to China on a work trip and had been chatting to someone on the net who wanted to meet me. He had a very poor opinion of women, which seemed pretty much the norm, and was out for total sexual enjoyment with a stranger. As much as it seemed exciting to chat to a stranger I still couldn't get my head round the fact that these men just wanted one night stands and no string fun.

I knew Mahmoud had always been faithful for whatever reason and he always used to say I am not like most men "99 per cent of men think with the dicks" Perhaps he had a point. I started to ponder. Men sexualized everything. They thought about sex more often than women. There was this connection between the brain and their cock, that's why they need visual and mental stimulus to have an orgasm. Either by watching porn, chatting via the net, or looking at some page three bird. My dad had a whole heap of pictures of page three girls pinned up in the shed mostly of Samantha fox. Once they had had an orgasm they normally roll over and fall asleep. Most women on the other hand tend to need that emotional attachment before they can commit to a sexual relationship. We are able to orgasm again and again. I guess it's that whole thing about "women being from Venus and men from Mars". There are of course exceptions and I think in some ways I was more masculine when it came to having sex. I was a sex addict to some degree and I could disconnect myself from it that was unless of course I fell into dangerous territory, and that was to fall in love.

The more I chatted the more I started to despise men. I liked to wind them up to make them feel like they were special but the reality was that I was nothing more than using them to analyse the male psyche behind the safety of my internet connection. I made sure I never used a logon name that was recognizable. When I chatted to men I even used to make up other profiles in order to find out whether they just wanted sex or a relationship. Most of the time I had been chatting to these men without them knowing I was using a different alias. It was easy to catch them out and I did frequently just for the hell of it. I went through a real period of hating men and everything they stood for. These men only thought with their cocks. It was all about what was in it for them. I knew that many of them would wank over pictures of my bottom which kind of disgusted me in a way and I sought to make things right. I joked one day and said people will pay good money to wank over my pictures.

Eventually after wading through all the mindless drivel and chat I talked to an Italian man through one site. His name was Marcello. I have always had a fascination for men from overseas, its that romantic way they speak, the way they talk to you, the way when he called me "Bella" it kind of rolled off the tongue. O Marcello what a sweet man you were. You don't know how much you changed my life. We talked on the net he had this passion that I needed so much. He seemed different from the other ones I had chatted to before, so I had this halfhearted expectancy that I had found a possible partner, when the reality was that I had met him in some dating site that was aimed at sex. He lived and worked in Germany and we had this bizarre sexual chemistry that engulfed a huge range of thoughts and emotions most of them involving him and me possibly stepping into the world of domination with another woman. We talked for hours on the phone. He was handsome and charismatic. He arranged to fly into Stanstead to meet me. All fired up with passion we planned to make mad passionate love to each other. The day he arrived I waited nervously in the arrivals lounge. Longing to see the face of the man I had been speaking to for weeks on the phone and the net. When he arrived there was this huge disappointment when I finally set eyes on him. The photograph I had been sent was about 10 years old. He was about 30 pounds heavier and he wasn't the Marcello I had imagined from the long phone conversations we had prior to meeting. I drove him back to the hotel where he was staying. And we talked and talked. There was no chemistry no passion and I felt disappointed that I had had this image of someone only to be disappointed. We spend the night sleeping next to each other back to back. No kissing, no intimacy and no sex

After he went back to Germany I asked him why he hadn't tried to sleep with me like all the others. He said he saw a vulnerability in me and although he had the impression when he first spoke to me on the phone that I was this sexually liberated woman, that was able to have non committal sex with a stranger, he saw that side of me that had been hurt and used in the past and didn't want to take advantage of that. Part of me was relieved because I didn't want to be having sex with someone just for the sake of it. I realized that night that the Internet dating was not for me. I wanted to have the romance again I wanted to meet a man in a normal way. I wanted to bump into him in a supermarket or over a drink in the pub. I didn't want to be introduced to a man who's first impression of me was my bum. It was weird and self destructive in some ways. Why didn't I just go out like everyone else why, was I still intrigued by this cyber world that had only brought me disappointment?

However for some reason, I continued nonetheless with my distraction of Internet chat for a while longer. Chatting online and then discarding them like some useless user. I thought that I could find some way of writing about the pitfalls of Internet dating from an experiential point of view. I wanted to show the world what a sad demoralizing place the Internet could be so I started to write a book. For my research, I became more daring, so I placed adverts, some of them totally outrageous, just for the hell of it, just to see what kind of a reaction I would provoke from these sad cheating men that were trawling the net. I even used to put a picture of my arse on the profiles I used. It was almost like saying, "kiss my arse". I imagined there were so many men jerking or wanking off at this picture of a bottom that could have been a man or some ugly monstrous woman. I thought how sad they were to be contacting me and I was even sadder to correspond back with them. The more I played with their minds the more I gained control and the more I spoke to them on the phone the more I realized I didn't want to be playing sexual games with strangers. I felt comfortable in the comfort zone of my own pc until one when I met a hacker metaphorically speaking. I had already begun to write my book with all the replies I had received from various men. Some of them were interesting, some of them very disgusting and totally demoralizing. I had an account with hotmail and disguised it under the name of open-minded something or other. I had hundreds of emails all from total strangers saying how they wanted to meet the woman with the "bum".

I never showed my face on the net. Started to file them in my inbox and often people would add themselves to my messenger when I logged on to chat. One day a man added himself to my messenger account. I think I went under the name of "well rounded bum" or something similar. He wanted to talk to me and I wasn't in the mood to chat. I had received a nice email from a young guy who seemed pleasant enough; different from the normal "I want to fuck your arse" type emails I received. The next day I received the same email from the other man who had added me to messenger. I copied the email to the original guy and said "I think someone has taken your words and copied them." It turned out that the "hacker" as I was soon to call him had logged randomly into someone's email account and read their emails taken their address and randomly approached me. I was online writing my book busy typing away when I decided to take a break and have a coffee. When I came back to log into my email account I found that I had been hacked into. He had changed my password while I was downstairs in the kitchen. There is a way of changing your password on hotmail and because I was tired I thought I would go and reset my password. He had changed my password to "Shyone is a big fat whore". My skin crawled when I realized he had gone into my email account and read all of these replies I had as research for my book. I mailed him back and said please don't do this then I received a dreadful awakening. He mailed me and said he had managed to hack into my email accounts. I always kept my own personal email account separate from the one I used for Internet research purposes.

I spent nights deleting every trace of my existence from my personal email accounts to my friends and family and backtracking so that he couldn't access anything. I decided the only action was to call the police. How would I explain why I had been hacked into? Would I have to explain that I had decided to write a book on internet dating? He sent me an email saying he was going to track me down and find me and kill me. It was like my whole personal space had been invaded. There was I playing this stupid mind games with stupid men on the net and now I'd been caught. I managed to salvage what I could of the research material I had gathered up over many months. The following day a bombshell was dropped. He had taken my contacts lists, which included a girl called sally who I had been talking to. He added himself to her list of contacts and managed to manoeuvre his way into her PC and hack into her customer database as she worked from home. She had no firewall or protection from attack and he wiped out her customer database overnight causing nearly 20 thousand pounds worth of lost business.

Rose Budworth Levine

The person in question was a woman called Sally. She was a bisexual woman who had her own business running as a travel agent. She had her own fair share of disastrous relationships. One included finding out that her boyfriend was a closet transvestite so she had decided to get her revenge on him by placing an ad in the local paper running it as a competition. She checked all the legal documentation before running it and it was basically a 'guess who this competition whereby someone had to phone and name that man.' Sweet revenge how delicious is was. How I wanted to be strong enough to have done 'that' over the years.

She was a very overbearing woman, loud and forceful but the hidden desires she had, was to be gangbanged. She had mailed me saying how she thought my profile was great and that she admired me as a woman. I think my profile, which changed from time to time, said something along the lines of 'Voluptuous woman not looking for anyone at the moment but interested to talk to couples about swinging. If I was to have an ideal man he would be tall, dark handsome with a huge tongue. He needs to be witty charming and above all rich, preferably a millionaire. If you not fit that description then you can kiss my arse LOLOLOL'. We met for drinks on a couple of occasions. She was a large woman, strict non-smoker who had lost complete control of herself and her dignity. She came across as very well presented, but the reality was she was lost in self-loathing and a large voluptuous body that she hated. She fantasized about being fucked by strangers and mentioned it in passing conversation. I said "I'll organize it for you". Much to my surprise she decided to take me up on the offer and I then proceeded to place an advert on a swingers site looking for half a dozen men (seemed like a nice rounded figure) to fuck a BBW women in a hotel. How outrageous I thought, and how on earth was I going to find these men.

Sally was very particular about what they should look like how they presented themselves and how she wanted this role acted out. She wanted to be blindfolded throughout and she wanted them all to be clean-shaven non smokers around 6 feet tall. I phoned a friend that I knew who told me about a hotel and placed an ad on some swinger's site. I didn't get many replies and I was surprised because I'd had so many replies to adverts I'd placed in the past for myself and had not followed through. So for a minute I thought on my feet. I had all these email addresses of guys that had wanted to meet me and I knew they were just looking for sex so I emailed them one by one and said they had chatted to me before on the net. I hadn't wanted to meet them but I had this friend that wanted to be fucked and gangbanged. I described her and arranged for 6 total strangers to come into a hotel room and get them to fuck her.

There she was stockings and Basque, legs spread on the bed blindfolded while this string of men entered the room. The first man to enter seemed to be ok so I confided in him how nervous I was at organizing such an event and he seemed to be a dab hand at these things. God forbid! I thought to myself, do men do this, go fuck a woman, one after its just like a piece of meat. While she lay on the bed I whispered in the bathroom explaining to each one at a time what was going to happen. I had no idea what was going to happen. What if she freaked out? What if she took off her blindfold and realized that these guys weren't all six foot hunks… and and and… my mind raced.

I kept opening the door and closing it so she had no concept of how many men were actually in the room. Was there five, 10, 20 who knows. She became more and more excited as I led each one into the main room. I was scared and excited. Most of these men were all men that had planned on meeting me initially and I hadn't reciprocated. Would they try to fuck me too or would I be able to keep control of the situation. I explained to them that I was not any part of what was going to happen and that I was certainly not the woman they were going to fuck and laughed hysterically, more out of nervousness. I stood next to the bed while each of them took turns to caress and touch this woman who was my friend, lying helpless on the bed with 6 total strangers touching every part of her body. She had been very specific about not wanting to have any of their cum on her and the next thing I new I was telling this woman what to do. I thought to myself how vulnerable she looked as she lay there helplessly doing nothing while they took turns to lick and suck and finger her pussy. Each one taking turns to push their hard cocks into her eager mouth. But at the same time she was enjoying every minute of it. "Now suck their cock I said". She proceeded to suck each one, one after another. In between multiple orgasms when each man eagerly sucked on her moist pussy. She then turned over and spread her legs blindfold still in place which each of them took turns to fuck her. At the same time she was sucking on another guys cock whilst she was being fucked and screaming with pleasure. At one point she was so overwhelmed with orgasm I had to put my hand over her mouth for fear of the rest of the hotel finding out what we doing in this room. One of the guys who had turned up decided to mop her sweaty body with a towel and rolled it up into an origami style bunny rabbit making motions as if it was going to fuck her too. I had to put my hand over my mouth and walk out for a brief moment. It all seemed so surreal. I wanted to laugh but at the same time the adrenalin of having all these guys under my control including my friend was amazing. The most surreal part was that this guy was about 5' 2" and had made her sequel more than the others. It was that whole image thing of these total handsome strangers fucking her that got her so excited.

After most of them left I felt this strange sense of empowerment how I was able to direct something so bizarre and feel so in control. I enjoyed the buzz that I got from knowing that these had all originally wanted to fuck me, but they couldn't and that power was overwhelming. It was shortly after that that I decided never to sleep with a man again. I wanted it to be different from this picture I had in my head of mindless surreal fucking. I wanted to make love to a man not just be some sex object and at that point I lost all respect for men in general. I realized that none of this was about me much as I wanted that power to be able to say no. The reality was it didn't matter who these men were fucking. It would, could have been a blow up doll just wanting a fuck and I was glad that wasn't me laying there in some hotel room.

After they left she took off her blindfold and we talked about what had happened. She explained that the one who had made her feel the most excited was the 5' 2" guy with the bunny ears origami rabbit, who just so happened to be a smoker, as well, and I had made him eat gum so his breath didn't smell. We went for a meal after and she said it was the most amazing thing that had happened to her. She said she never felt such excitement and mostly from the lack of control she had over her environment. In her own life she was so controlling she said she felt like a different woman and that the total escapism was what excited her.

INTIMATE ENCOUNTERS

6 - THREE INTO TWO DOESN'T GO

I had always had a fantasy about being with another woman. Part of it stemmed from an initial encounter I had with an old friend. I had always travelled around the world and during that time I made some good friends. One of them was a girl from Australia a very petite looking princess that had an almost child like figure. I was friends with her brother Richard who was gay and we used to go out together mostly to get drunk. I guess I was about twenty-one when I met her. We had been drinking for most of the evening and innocently ended up in bed together kissing and fondling. I wanted to see what it would feel like to taste a woman so I slowly started to undress her and slip off her underwear. She had an almost pubescent type figure, no breasts to speak of and as I fumbled away with my tongue I realized there was no response from her. It tainted the way I felt about bi-sexual relationships and I never really thought about it again until my mid thirties.

I started to talk to a Belgian girl via email. A beautiful voluptuous brunette with long flowing dark curly hair and the most amazing green eyes you could imagine. She shared the same birthday as me and there was a naivety in me, almost narcissistic that attracted me to her. She was twenty-one and her name was Anais and she was what I imagined myself to have been at twenty-one. She carried all the same insecurities as I did at that age. But she had the most amazing depth of character that I was drawn to. She was prone to depression and had an almost incestuous type relationship with her father as her younger brother had died when she was very young and she was the sole member of the family. She had been bought up a strict catholic girl and had a long term boyfriend who wanted to introduce her into the world of swinging. She had met several men but her passion was women. She had a very dominant demeanour. You could just feel the power as she entered the room but at the same time this almost childlike insecurity that wanted to be nurtured. She mentioned on many occasions that she wanted to be a dominatrix and we laughed so many times about how much fun it would be. We started to look at dungeon premises in London and planned how we would rule the world and become these two almost mother and child like doms. How we would take the fetish world by storm and be the most incredible BBW dominatrix duo. I had already started to do my homework looking at websites and discussing how we were going to work together and we talked daily about our plans and how we were going to start a business together. She was such a fragile woman in such a strong sexy voluptuous body. The first time we made love to each other she was like a submissive child. She wanted so much to please me and I remember the first time she gave me oral sex. She said to me in the 'most sexy' French accent. Please Rose, I want you to sit on my face and cum for me." "There is nothing more I want to do than pleasure you". Such a contrast from the discussions we had earlier that day about dominating men and how she had this overwhelming urge to fuck a man with a strap on.

During our relationship I had been seeing a man by the name of John. He was a bad boy, tattoos all over the place. I was never even sure his name was actually John, but I had met him through a friend. I had arranged to meet my friend called Jenny who was a swinger. I was fascinated by them to be honest, and they were making excellent research material for my book. As much as I was intrigued by the lifestyle I could never get my head round the endless encounters Jenny had with men. She would often fuck one after another week in week out, an endless sea of faces just there waiting to fuck her and then be on their way. Jenny was disabled. She had three slipped discs from being beaten senseless by a client whilst working as a probation officer. She had the most amazing blue eyes and long soft auburn hair. In contrast to her disability where she could not walk for more than a couple of hundred yards her legs were beautiful. She had previously been a leg model for a big company that sold tights. Those beautiful legs that couldn't even carry her around could manage to wrap themselves around a man's thighs easy enough. Those beautiful legs that she would spread for the endless men that wanted to fuck her time and again.

We had arranged on that night to go for a social evening at a swingers club. She introduced me to a couple that were friends of hers and we sat in the pub talking. Next to her was one of her new "prospectives". She used to interview them almost in a cold calculating way to see if they were viable to fuck her. This man was sitting there, pierced eyebrow, and I looked at him and thought "there was this animal magnetism that I couldn't fathom." I kept looking at him and couldn't divert my eyes. That evening, we all left the pub and I was to take Jenny to this club. So we said our goodbyes and I drove with her and John to the club. He had to work that night and said if we wanted to call later after we left the club. I walked up to the entrance. Jenny, her walking stick in hand, looked all glammed up and ready to fuck everything in site. It was never my way to do that. I used to go to the clubs as the observer. I was fascinated by the fact that total strangers could go into a room and undress and then have sex with each other in a way that was hedonistic and primal. I remember being an onlooker where there was this revolving table that could hold about 12 bodies. Each woman lined up with their legs spread, all the men standing around ready to fuck each woman in turn. I remember thinking how disgusted I felt especially as none of them seemed to have any idea about safe sex but there was this excitement in watching what was purely primal.

That night jenny and I were to go to the club she walked through the door and the receptions asked if she was a member. She said no, and mentioned that she had a problem with her disability and would it be ok for her to go into the club, but at some point she would need carrying up the stairs. There were two friends waiting for her in the doorway. An old guy that looked to be around sixty was with this nymphet type young woman with plump breasts as his partner. What kind if partnership was that all about? Here was an incestuous relationship between some old pervert and a young nubile woman who looked young enough to be my daughter. The club decided not to let Jenny in on this occasion because of her disability. She kicked up a fuss and made herself out to be a victim of discrimination but then that's what she always did. Jenny was victim of her own self-destruction, destroying herself by this endless tirade of men one after another. Taking what was theirs for the taking and destroying every part of her self esteem as they went along. I had talked to her on many occasions saying that swinging was not a lifestyle for anyone and that it would only be a matter of time before she became attached to someone. You can't always have sexual encounters with anyone without there being that special bond, and I was learning that more and more as time went on.

We sat in the pub for sometime and it was late. I suggested we called her friend John, part of me being very selfish for wanting to see him again. I remember Jenny saying "he wont come because he is working" and me saying "no he'll come because he is a man!." I wanted to tease and wind him up so we invited him to the hotel. made him sit on the bed and watch while I caressed and touched Jenny's delicate body. There was no intimate contact as we didn't have that kind of a relationship but the power I felt watching him watch us as we touch and kissed was amazing. It was after that evening that I started seeing him.

We dated for a few months during which time I had expressed my desires to have a proper intimate relationship with another woman and that woman was Anais. The beautiful Amazonian goddess who I had been seeing who had bought out a whole new sexual side to me. John on the other hand was dangerous, a real bad boy. We had grown to understand each other during the months we were together. He had obsessive-compulsive disorder bought on by the death of his longterm girlfriend. He never attached himself to anyone and I was grateful for the time we spent together. We would chat and laugh and get high and have great sex and then I would wind him up again as I always did about his fantasy of being with two women. He had been living with his girlfriend for a number of years.

It was as he described the perfect romance before his detachment of feelings towards women. He was never meant to be with another woman as far as I could see. He had been fishing one night and came answered his phone early morning expecting his girlfriend to call but it was her sister calling him. That night his girlfriend had died in her sleep aged 32 years old, of a heart attack whilst he had been out fishing. What a tragic story and he was never to get over it. I knew that there would not be a loving relationship with this man whilst his heart was still attached to his girlfriend but in my own warped twisted sense I wanted to make things right for him. I Talked to him one night and suggested he should meet my friend Anais. I said he would love her and that she was a young version of me. She was very sexy and very appealing and very childlike. Of course he was a man and he would delight at the thought of meeting me and her together. I spoke to Anais and said I wanted to introduce her to my boyfriend. She was very excited at the prospect. I warned her that he was a bad boy and that I would never attach myself to him because if I did I would only end up breaking my heart but I said he had a raw sexuality that needed exploring.

We arranged to meet one evening and we politely chatted and drank and got very stoned. We ended up in a hopeless pile of bodies on the bed each taking turns to pleasure each other. I remember looking deep into Anais eyes while she was licking my pussy and being fucked from behind by John. She had this look of the devil in her and that laugh. It was a moment that came from pure lust. That night he left and I fell asleep on the bed next to Anais and she stayed for a couple of days longer. We went, we shopped, we talked. It was the one time I thought I may be able to live with a woman but I knew that that was something that was never going to happen.

I had arranged to see her the following week and for some reason I had this gut feeling that she wouldn't turn up. We always chatted on the net on Messenger or Yahoo and it never occurred to me that she would fall for someone, but then again she was a younger version of me with that yearning that seems so strong with youth. I had a worried call from her boyfriend that night. Her phone was off and she had disappeared. What transpired was that she had arranged to see John a few days later. She had fallen in love with him as her boyfriend put it and they had run off to the coast. He then explained her dark side to me saying she had been very immature with men was prone to suicidal thoughts and although he had been her partner for many years she had the overwhelming desire to find that "bad boy" who just happened to be John.

I emailed her and warned her that he wasn't good for her. He was very self destructive and I spoke to him to and he explained that it was just a fling, as it been with me and there no intention of getting involved with her. It was a weird kind of surreal situation whereby two people I had been with so intimately were to disappear from my life. To this day I never knew what happened to Anais. I believe she went back to Belgium and John, well, he is just drifting along in his aimless existence hoping his girlfriend might reappear one day.

INTIMATE ENCOUNTERS

7 - THE POWER OF A WOMAN

So I never did end up become a dominatrix with Anais. I guess we were never destined to be that all consuming duo of Amazonian goddesses. I decided that from that point on I never wanted to have sex with a man again unless it was special. I had done my experimenting and thought the only way forward for me to gain control was to start dominating. I was celibate from the minute I started; I remained celibate for 1 year, apart from a brief fling and then another year after that. I decided to dominate on my own initially from hotels as I had no premises to work from. There was one place in East London that Anais had pointed out and I was looking into working from there.

The first encounter I had was with a Spanish man who was into body worship and feet. I met him at his hotel. I remember going into his room and him saying that the minute we entered we would be in character. Role-play, character, some strange terminology I had never heard of. As we entered the room I told him to get himself undressed and I would go into the bathroom. I came out of the bathroom dressed in a long black coat and high heels. Underneath I wore stockings and a purple taffeta Basque. It wasn't particular fetish or dome but I felt powerful. There was this small man around 5' 4" kneeling beneath me naked and ready to do as I told him. I walked across the room with a dignified grace and told him to kneel down and kiss my feet. It was the

87

first time I was to hear the words uttered "yes mistress". Then I proceeded to make him kiss my bottom. As I was instructing him to do it in the manner I wanted I remember thinking he had found it difficult to follow directions when arriving at the hotel. So as his tongue wandered aimlessly towards the cleft of my bottom I turned my head and said "Kiss my bottom, and kiss every part of it so you understand exactly how to please me. You need to follow my instructions. I do hope your skills as a slave are better than your skills of navigation" "your not very good with directions are you slave?" He giggled and said "yes Mistress"

My second encounter was with a pilot. It wasn't on a professional basis. I knew I was going to become a good dominatrix but I had so much to learn and I didn't have the confidence to pull off a professional encounter. I had chatted to this guy on Alt. He was a very handsome striking man who worked for the RAF as a pilot. I guess during his working life he was so in control he wanted to have that control taken away from him and he was on the face of it submissive. He lived in a beautiful house in Norfolk and I was invited down for the weekend to play. We had a few drinks to break the ice whilst I sat in his grand lounge in front of a roaring fireplace. The same fireplace I had seen in the background of a picture he had mailed me of him dressed totally in rubber and stockings and heels. He made a polite excuse and then disappeared upstairs. When he came down he had this huge suitcase of gadgets. Unbelievable things I had never seen before, gags, blindfolds, harnesses, hoods, masks, dildos. There must have been a mini dungeon all in one bag. I started to panic, what was I thinking how I could I dominate a man that new more about this than me. I had read things on the web and was starting to understand the language used. It was like a whole new learning process for me. I was a quick learner and I had to think fast on my feet. We talked for sometime before meeting and his interests were strap-on training. God forbid the only time I had stuck my fingers up a man's arse was when I was married and my ex husband used to enjoy the sensation as I gave him his usual blow job.

Lube in hand I started to finger his arse. As this tall statuesque man was kneeling on the floor of his lounge with his legs spread eagerly awaiting me to finger his arse. He had some poppers in his hand and started to sniff them and then each time as more fingers probed he asked me to put more into his expanding bottom. I started to feel the muscles relax as the poppers started to work and before I knew it and half a bottle of lube later I had my fist in his bottom. I wasn't really sure how I felt. There was this very confident strong man totally giving himself up to a woman in the most perverse fashion letting her fist his arse. I fisted him and he wanked himself all over the carpet. That was an interesting introduction to strap on training as I was soon to find out later what strap on actually meant.

As time went on I needed to find premises to work. I had my website all ready to go then I began to get cold feet. I was still seeing Jenny, she was getting more poorly by the minute her legs were weak. Her bladder was paralysed and the only way she could go to the bathroom was to press her bladder. I felt sorry for her, She was still swinging and as much as I tried to persuade her that this was going to destroy her life I wanted to help, so I suggested she work with me. I told her I would set up a joint website and we could work together. We could go and use the dungeon in London and make double appointments. At first the appointments came trickling in. She lived a couple of hours north of me so she would drive down and we would go to London for the day and work. The money helped her a lot as she was about to lose her home and her daughter. I started to enjoy the domination, I liked the power I got from seeing men at my feet however Jenny bless her, didn't have a dominant bone in her body.

She was a victim and that's what split us apart. One day she decided to meet a guy off the net that she had never spoken to albeit a brief telephone conversation. She had a beautiful daughter that was the same age as my son and she decided to take this total stranger into her house and let him fuck her. Her daughter was asleep upstairs in the bedroom. I was so disappointed in her that she had so little self esteem that she could let her sexual life interfere with her family and I tried to talk to her. We argued and I said she was a victim and that I could no longer work with her. More and more I was doing sessions with her and being told off in session for being too mean to the submissive when the reality was that that's what they wanted. That total submission, the total lack of control. I tried to explain to her that that's what these men were paying for. Paying for us to take away the control but she could never understand how any man could enjoy pain. I began to enjoy Cock ball torture. I still can't fathom out why I enjoyed it so much. I think it stemmed from the fact that there was this helpless man with an erection who was willing to let you torture his cock and balls. She found it very disturbing.

We came back one day from the station and I was tired because she needed looking after, wanted to help but she wasn't helping herself. I wanted to give her the empowerment I felt I was getting. She phoned me when she got home and said she had slept with three men that week. She was back swinging again and one of the guys she had met had threatened to beat her but she was still seeing him. Her previous relationships had been very destructive. She also had cervical cancer probably as a result of the amount of men she had slept with and was still having a succession of sexual encounters even though her health was at risk. I told her she was a victim and that if she didn't help herself I couldn't work with her anymore. She went mad and said she never wanted to see me again, she wrote me a disgusting email saying how I had taken her livelihood away from despite the fact that she hated working as a dominatrix. She said I had used her victim status against her because of her injury.   I tried to explain that the victim was referring to her not her disability.

We parted company and I started to work alone. It was a scary feeling having to do it professionally even though I had done it on many occasions before I'd started to work with Jenny. I was travelling to and from London a couple of days a week and although some of the sessions I did seemed amateurish I was starting to feel my way in the world of domination.

I had always had a fascination for total empowerment by sitting on a man's face. Maybe part of that stemmed from the fact that my husband had not "gone down there for the last 15 years" That feeling that they were just some worthless tongue to be used for my pleasure, but at the same time knowing that should I decide I could crush their face with my large voluptuous bottom, I could do so. Part of the thrill of domination was that men sexualized everything ultimately. It was the denial that really sparked me. The fact that they couldn't have what they wanted. For example if they wanted to worship my pussy I wanted them to kiss my ass instead. Making them feel they were not worthy. If they wanted to have an orgasm I wanted to deny them it. I had been working in London and eventually bought my own premises nearer to home.   It had been a really difficult couple of months as I had been letting the dungeon to a full-time in-house slave who had contacted me through and internet site. He had been on the scene for a few years and his name was Damien. He was in his fifties and I knew of him through my ex husband and the underground dance scene. I had organized a psychedelic trance parties many years ago in an old warehouse in East London with his brother. So we shared the same interests in music. He was quite heavily into the scene and did lighting shows for a number of different groups. He wanted to live a 24/7 lifestyle and stay at the dungeon as a totally feminized slut who I could use and abuse as I saw fit. Of course the fantasy and reality are two quite different things. He even talked about eating shit, one of my other big no no's, so one day I remember doing a big dump on the loo the first time I met him on purpose to test him out. It knocked that fantasy on the head because it stank terrible. I actually cared about my subs and some of the things they wanted to do were outrageous. So I suggested that instead of going full on 24/7 it might be an idea to take things slowly. He had wanted to take a complete year out and quit from his part-time work and go straight into being a slut full-time. I knew there was something not quite right so I encouraged him to carry on doing the work and, seeing his friends from time to time and break him in slowly.

It's the one saving grace I have, is an understanding of people. I always like to think I am a good judge of character. Sometimes it takes a while for the penny to drop but eventually I get there. At first things were fine he was very good about keeping the place clean and tidy almost to the point of obsession. I would do my sessions and he would have a chat when I came over. Even went to a party with him that he had arranged. But things got worse, his behaviour becoming more and more erratic. He had a drug habit I hadn't known about until he moved in. He was smoking pot every single day, how much I have no idea. His mood swings were so unpredictable. One minute tearful and wanting to be looked after telling me his life story how he had had a terrible childhood, and how he was on long term sick for post traumatic stress having seen one of his mates boiled alive on a merchant sea trip.

I felt sorry for him but I was starting to be scared to go to work. When I tried to talk to him about things he would stick his fingers in his ears and say things like "nah nah nah I can't hear you, I am not listening to you". I believe he was either bipolar or schizophrenic, probably triggered off by years and years of emotional problems and drug abuse. I was very gentle with him and thankfully my gut instinct had been right and I never played with him or introduced him to any clients. He said he felt like a prisoner and that all the things he thought he wanted to do had gone right out of his head. He was fighting with friends outside, behaving manically, not sleeping for hours on end. So when I went over to work he would be so angry because I would have to creep around doing my sessions while he slept. One time I called him to say I was going to be there to make sure it was ok for me to go and he didn't pick up the phone, so I called his mobile. He had left it downstairs and gone to pick up my call. He hit his head on the stairs and then called me screaming his head off telling me it was my entire fault... I called the client and met them for a drink in a local hotel apologising for not being able see them. Luckily a chance offer of a flat in the South coast came up and he moved out after three months.

During that time, I had been working for about a year on my own when I decided to branch out and met another dominatrix through work who had come for a session with her husband to celebrate their anniversary. They were late for their appointment and I had another client waiting to see me who had arrived early. The couple that came, she was Dom and he was sub. They had been living a sub Dom role for the past 10 years and he had a fantasy of being a 24/7 TV cuckold slut. From what I gathered from our conversations after the session he would do the housework, would laze around most of the day going off having her sun beds and painting her false fingernails and then she would abuse and humiliate him. He told me once in conversation that she wasn't a Dom from the beginning but he had introduced her and she was a good learner.

Her name was Shirley and on their anniversary she wanted to give her husband Martin a present to remember and had indicated in her prior emails that he would like to try forced Bi. So there I was one client late the other early so I had to think fast on my feet. I decided that the best option was to see all the clients together. So I led the single guy into the main dungeon area and took the couple into the back room. My plan was to session with the first guy and then to introduce the couple into the session later. I was anxious about Damian being downstairs as he had been acting strange the day before and was not speaking to me. I needed to earn some money as I had been avoiding working there for a few days. So putting my thinking cap on I created one of my many forced Bi sessions. I ordered him on his knees into the dungeon. The other slave tied up and told him "Get on your knees and suck his cock".

A few weeks later I had introduced Shirley to my web host and she was working as a professional dominatrix. I helped her to set up and gave her advice about how I dealt with clients on a professional basis, how to email them discuss on the phone, deal with the timewasters. It wasn't long before she was working and sessioning in my own dungeon and visiting me on a regular basis. She had two children one with dyslexia and the other with Asperger's syndrome. He was a sweet child in a little world of his own about the same age as my own son. But his emotions were a little mixed up. They visited once and wrecked my son's bedroom and the snooker table fell on top of the guinea pig that was in a cage underneath. I came running upstairs and Charlie was playing x box the other boys trying desperately to hold the table up when Charlie said "I like the Xbox more than I like guinea pigs"

We had this arrangement where my family thought I was in business with her doing accounting and she would come up for a couple of days a month. I had always wanted to do filming and start up a website putting my dominatrix talents on film and so she suggested that we start a site together. I was in debt and had no money to initiate a new site and she seemed to be keen to help. We started filming. Most of my slaves were happy to be on film. There was something narcissistic about them that they enjoyed the fact that thousands of other men would we downloading videos of them being dominated. They trusted me not to put their faces on my site if we had agreed so I did most of the work myself.

Shirley did little apart from come up and appear in the films. She made it clear that she hated her husband with a vengeance and that she found it disgusting that he was submissive and wanted to do forced Bi videos. He wanted to be in on everything but she liked the fact that she could get away from him. When she stayed he would call sometimes 60 times a day if she didn't answer the phone, she said he was Aspergers like her son. One day her son Charlie reported his father for beating him at school. The authorities were called in and she phoned up with no emotion. Charlie had lied about the abuse but because of his condition, she was so angry and she said I hope they take the little fucker away. That's when I realised something was wrong.

She had taken the boys bedroom away from them and started setting up a dungeon where she could session from home. I wasn't happy that she was working in an environment where her children might see. I was starting to get anxious and was very unhappy about doing all the work for the site and providing all of my subs for films so I confronted her one-day and said I wanted her to bring in some subs of her own. I needed space. She suffered from huge insecurities. Had spent years being overweight and then nearly seven stone with pills and had to have surgery remove the extra skin that was left. I too had been overweight and had stretch marks but I saw it as part of who I was. She bleached her hair, spent hours on treatments and wouldn't dare go out of the house without a ton of makeup on her face. Her husband Martin came from a rich posh family and was waiting for an inheritance. His own father had died of Alzheimer's and they were fighting for a 4 million pound inheritance, which would have ended up in trust for the children otherwise. When I confronted her about the site, she was angry. I was about to go on holiday with my children so we agreed to sort things out when we got back.

8 - OBSESSIVE LOVE

During the time that I was also a friend with Shirley I hadn't been seeing anyone for over two years and had not been in any kind of sexual relationship. One day I got a call from a guy asking for face sitting. I remember I was on my period at the time and couldn't take a booking so I decided to postpone. He said his name was Paul. I don't remember actually arranging another date specifically but I got a text the following week from him saying I am sorry I can't make my appointment today but would I give him some indication as to what I was going to do in session with him when he eventually came. I thought he's probably looking for wanking material, so being flippant I texted him back saying "I will blow your mind!" Within minutes I had a text back from him saying could he come that day. He arrived around 5 or 6 pm that day.

I was sitting in the front room having given him directions and he just breezed past the window. All I could think was oh my god. I'd been in that position before when I had first met Alex and Mahmoud it was that feeling you get that you cant describe like its your destiny to have met them. I thought I loved him from the minute I saw him but I realize now that I was just obsessed. He came into the room tall, attractive and floppy hair quite unshaven. He smelt of alcohol and was very nervous. I gestured him to sit down and put my hand on his and tried to calm his nerves. I then explained how I would do the session as I always did and gestured him to go upto the room. It had been a really hot day and I normally wore leather and high heels, but on this day I didn't feel the need to put on the mask and had joked earlier asking him if he had any preference to my clothing and he joked I could dominate him naked if I wanted. I ended up wearing a regular skirt and blouse and underneath I wore a simple g-string body stocking to hide my modesty. When I got into the room he was still very nervous and he said your not going to film me are you, I think the camera might have been on the side of the room. I just laughed and said of course not wondering how he could be so paranoid. One of the first things I got him to do was to kneel down and worship my bottom. I knew from that minute what he wanted and the whole session was electric and I believe I probably did blow his mind. Interestingly enough when I got to sit on his face I didn't come at all. He was all enthusiastic but no technique, but I knew just by his body language he enjoyed the sensation of being overpowered by my bum I wanted to kiss him throughout the whole session, I wanted to be more sensual and loving but I couldn't he was a client. After we finished I had this overwhelming urge to see him again. It's the first time I have wanted to see one of my clients even though I have had many who have wanted to see me. We sat in the kitchen having a coffee and chat and he explained that he possibly wanted a 24/7 relationship.

I knew he wasn't really submissive just experimenting; you got a feel for it after a while. I told him if he ever wanted to chat or have a drink outside of work he was more than welcome. He confessed that his name was not Paul but Dan which made me laugh, he didn't look anything like a Paul and Paul was the most common name subs used to phone when making appointments. A few days later I texted him. It was strange because during that week we talked and talked on the phone albeit he was so nervous he had to have a drink before he could pluck up the courage to talk to me. He seemed to put me on a pedestal and he was saying he was starting to miss me. I was thinking, "oh my god I have met some crazy alcoholic thats going to end up stalking me", and being the pathetic type of sub I despised so much in session. Little was I to know that I would end up being the pathetic submissive woman because he would destroy my character. I wanted a real man, someone who would make me feel like a woman. We stopped talking for a while and I decided I could not see him, then for some reason there was a breakthrough one day and we arranged to meet up. We slept with each other the first time we dated. It was the first time in years I didn't feel the need to cover up my body or dress in a certain way; it was the first time I felt like I could be myself.

We saw each other for a few months usually on his day off. He was so secretive and elusive, one minute showing a glimpse of his feelings and the next shutting me out. He would switch his phone off for days at a time or make arrangements to meet and then change his mind at the last minute. He suffered from extreme paranoia. We were supposed to go to a club with some friends a big fetish event in Surrey. He loved wearing a collar when we first sessioned together as client, so I had bought him a necklace to wear instead of the usual studded dog lead. He was so paranoid he thought that wearing a collar was some kind of secret code indicating his sexual orientation, which just made me laugh and laugh. We broke up a few weeks later for the first time and we were to break up again and again. I wrote him a long letter, one of many I would write asking him to come back. He would come back and say lets take things more slowly then within hours or days it was all full on again.

He worked as a DJ in the evenings a couple of nights a week. Those were the nights he would send me texts back and forth. None of which made too much sense to anyone else and most of which were a result of drugs or alcohol talking. He told me I was everything he ever wanted in a woman but he didn't know what to do with me. I always thought deep down it was the alcohol talking. I realized as time went on he had lots of issues, issues about his family, his work, his self-esteem. I had tried to help him with his problems and initially he seemed open to my advice saying, "I listen to every word Rose." But as time went on he seemed to see it as nagging and started to treat me with an arrogance that was so disconcerting. I remember one day driving up to his work with a bad back to deliver some records for him and tell him I wanted him to move in at some point with me and start over again. Maybe help him to realize his dreams and potential and allow him the freedom to start all over again, and maybe become a writer as he had said he always wanted to do. I just wanted him to think about things and stop destroying himself. But instead of thanking me for what I thought was a genuine gesture, he just thought I was imposing on his space and met me briefly for a few minutes giving me a look as if I was something on the bottom of his shoe.

My feelings of self-worth were rapidly diminishing. It was all made worse by the fact I was drowning in debt and my health was suffering as a result of all the stress I had. I was getting repetitive cluster migraines that would last for up to a week at a time. I had terrible self doubt and the fact that he kept running away again and again, then would come back into my life like a whirlwind and go out of it again just as quickly. He related to the world in a dynamic kind of impulsiveness. Even turning up on his day off would be down to whether he had got drunk or smashed the night before and if he could be bothered to turn up. He never wanted to make a decision and I think he always kept his options open. He never wanted to be slowed down by something as banal as being careful or committed and I don't thing he ever realized the kind of turmoil his actions generated. As much as I loved his free spirit I was starting to despise him for his selfishness.

Rose Budworth Levine

I had to stop seeing him for my own sanity. I was slipping into depression which I have suffered on and off for many years. In addition I had so many problems to deal with, debt, family crisis, dom burnout. His actions were totally demoralizing me, I would end up feeling like I had done something wrong and being even more paranoid than he was. The more he treated me the way he did the more I chased him and then pushed him away as fast as I could and then I would chase him again. He kept saying to me, open up to him, and I had opened up to him so much I had released all the demons I had been hiding for years. He made me feel so vulnerable and helpless in the end when in fact I was generally strong and motivated before I met him. I felt like he had opened me up like one of the books he always liked to read. He picked out the interesting parts that he wanted and then got bored and decided to leave me on the side for someone else to read. As much as I opened up he was a closed book. I had no idea of his surname for months, I didn't know where he lived, I didn't have a home phone number, and I had never met any of his friends. And even the times when I had to go drop letters at his work I had the feeling he always had something to hide from me.

I decided I couldn't see him until I had sorted out my problems. He was the one thing that had bought a smile to my face for a few months but he was destroying me. I took a letter up to his work to tell him, lets just see what happens in January. I met him briefly for five minutes in the

INTIMATE ENCOUNTERS

alleyway of the shopping centre. He was in a hurry to get back to work. I wanted to say to him there and then, I am dying Dan. I didn't even want to get out of bed in the mornings I was so depressed. Instead I had put some makeup on and make my hair nice and told him I was fine. I drove home and cried all the way and then again the next day. On the Tuesday my mother told me she had a lump in her breast. I thought the one person I could call would be Dan because he was going through some problems with his father who was dying. I thought he would understand. As I sobbed on the phone all he could say was how he would get into trouble for me calling him at work. He promised to call and of course that call never came. I put the phone down sobbing again wishing I had never picked up and phone and called him. I sobbed for another two days, not even getting out of bed apart from dropping the kids off at school. Then on the Friday morning I woke up with the overwhelming urge to end my life. It was the third or fourth time in as many months I had felt this way. I was later to find out it was the day George Best died. I had to go to the dungeon to meet one of my subs that was fixing the electricity for me. We had a nice friendly chat and then I cleared out all the paperwork in the dungeon making sure everything was in order as I had planned to go home and then drop off any paperwork there.

I spent the rest of the day writing suicide letters. I wrote, one to my kids, one to my best friend asking them to clear out the dungeon, one to Dan and one to another slave called H.   I arranged for the children to stop over at friends and family that night.   I was going to stop in a hotel and fill my stomach with alcohol and paracetamol, at least that way I wouldn't have to face the pain I was feeling. I even called my ex husband and told him he would have to take care of the children because I wasn't well. Well I wasn't well I was depressed and hurting in a way I couldn't explain to anyone.   All I needed was a kind word from Dan at least that's what I thought. He promised to call earlier in the week. He always promised to call and never did.   Something happened that day that made me change my mind. I had emailed a psychic woman and sent her a desperate email saying I was going to take my own life. I was sitting alone at the computer when she mailed me back and suggested I call her. She offered to listen to me without any judgement. I poured everything out to her, how I had had two failed marriages, how I had overcome my Chrohns disease over the past few years, how I had suffered from chronic recurring migraines that totally dilapidated me over a period of days every month. I told her about Dan, about my problems with my daughter and explained about the domination and how difficult it was to keep up such a brave face all the time when I was drowning in debt. She tried to alleviate my fears and convince me, saying how all my loved ones would feel if I wasn't around any more. I sobbed again and again and in the end just fell asleep from sheer exhaustion.

INTIMATE ENCOUNTERS

The following day my best friend Adam came round to try and cheer me up. In the afternoon I arranged to take my son window-shopping as Christmas was approaching. I spotted my youngest brother and his wife walking towards us. He had had a troubled teenage life and left home late in life. He was mollycoddled by my mother and ended up marrying, what turned out to be almost another mother figure. The whole family had fallen out over his desire to distance himself from us all. We talked politely for a few minutes and then he walked off towards the main part of the shopping centre. I was so angry with him for treating me like a stranger. I wanted to tell him how selfish he was and that he should make an effort to find out what the family were doing. I wanted to tell him his mother was going to die soon and I wanted to shout at him and tell him I used to change his nappies when he was a baby and how could he treat me the way he did. Instead I just walked away with my son Francis holding my hand. I wandered around for a while with him to the toyshop to buy some matchbox cars. When we walked back I went past the same chain of shops where Dan worked. I looked in there and saw my brother John and his wife at the counter. I wanted to run into the shop and put my arms round him and tell him how much I loved and missed him then for a brief second I thought perhaps I will start up a conversation with him as he worked in Birmingham. I wanted to tell him I had met this guy I was so happy to be with who worked in the same company in Birmingham. I was confused and angry and hurt and I had to hide the tears again from my son.

Then the penny dropped as I walked home hand-in-hand with my son. He looked up at me and said "why are you so sad mummy?" I said "oh just everything, money, seeing my brother again". He said "You were always happy when you were seeing Dan" I smiled and said "I Know". "in fact you were the happiest I have seen you in ages" he said." I thought for a minute and then realized that happiness for me would only ever come in brief moments during my life.

So there I was the day before contemplating suicide and trying to explain to a nobody who worked in a store and who didn't give one second thought to the emotional turmoil he had created, by just being elusive and not being brave enough to face up to the fact that a bit of kindness would have gone such a long way. I realized I despised his selfishness and had a horrible vision of him dying the same death as George Best because the alcohol would always mean more to him that my friendship.

But who was I to judge him I would probably die a miserable death myself for being the dominatrix, the slut buggerer, the forced bi specialist that would make grown men do unthinkable things by sucking each other off, the humiliatrix who would make men weak at the knees with her power by forcing them to stick their tongue up my bottom hole and clean it, the woman who could stick cigarettes stubs out on a mans chest while cumming all over his face. I had been on the PC the night before and did a test on the net. It was called "Dante's Inferno Test". Basically a test where it asked you a number of questions and then gave you an answer as to what level of hell you were at. The reply I got was this: 'Level 2: You have come to a place mute of all light, where the wind bellows as the sea does in a tempest. This is the realm where the lustful spend eternity. Here, sinners are blown around endlessly by the unforgiving winds of unquenchable desire as punishment for their transgressions. The infernal hurricane that never rests hurtles the spirits onward in its rapine, whirling them round, and smiting, it molests them. You have betrayed reason at the behest of your appetite for pleasure, and so here you are doomed to remain. Cleopatra and Helen of Troy are two that share in your fate.' I Laughed and laughed and laughed!

The following day I had a booking it was a Sunday. I never normally work on a Sunday but money was even tighter than normal. I had been ill the previous week with one of my many migraines and I had spoken to this man before on a number of occasions. He was from Belgium and was driving up from Dorset for the day. I knew he would turn up; you kind of get a feel for it after a while. His scenario was that he wanted to be caught asleep by his auntie and be punished for looking up my skirt. The punishment would be in the form of face sitting, bottom worship and strap-on-play.

I met him at the dungeon at the allotted time, we had a brief chat and then I was off into role-play. I really wasn't in the mood to work, least of all sit on some guys face for a couple of hours. Nonetheless I did what I had to do. All the time I was thinking about Dan and how he had first come to see me for face sitting. This guy's body reaction was just the same, the wriggling and squirming whilst I sat on his face. The excitement when as I dominated him. He stayed for 2 hours and I finished him off with a golden shower. He showered and left. After he went tears began to well up in my eyes again. Why was I doing this godforsaken job, it all seemed ok when I was seeing Dan, in fact the way he talked about it and admired what I was doing it all seemed right? I knew Dan got excited at the thought of me dominating other men but part of the attraction for me to see him was that he was a normal everyday bloke. I didn't want a guy that would rather get pissed up, that wanted to go down the pub and be with his mates. I didn't want a guy that would rather watch cricket than spend time with or even take a call from me. I wanted to be that normal woman, wanted to have vanilla sex, wanted to curl up next to the person I loved and wake up in the morning without the need to be dominant all the time. I wanted to be made love too, be kissed and touched and caressed and not be the object of someone's fetish for once. I wanted someone to tell me everything would be ok, I would be able to pay my debts off in time, it was ok for me to cry and be a woman. I wanted someone to tell my darkest secrets and fears and for them to listen. But I didn't have any of that instead I had 200 pounds in my pocket which would go fractionally towards paying off my huge debts. And I had a dungeon full of whips and paddles and butt plugs and fetish gear.

I had a phone call that evening from a young woman. She had seen my website and wanted some advice about becoming a dominatrix. She was twenty-two. I asked her why she wanted to work as a Dom and she said mainly because she had debts and she wanted to pay her way through university. She explained that she wanted to do cock-ball torture and ball-busting and would be happy hurting men because she didn't like the male species very much. She had had a string of disastrous relationships, which had left her hating men in general. We had a long discussion and I explained that being a Dom wasn't all it was made out to be, ok the money was good, but how would she feel if she had such contempt for men now. If for example, she realized that the majority of men that came through my door wanted to be dressed as a woman, many were afraid of their own sexuality and wanted women to fuck their arses instead of a man. Many were even closet gays not in touch with their real feelings and wanted to give oral sex to another man or fuck them, but wrap it up all up domination. I asked her how would that cloud her vision, how would that taint her perception of men even more. Then I explained about the time-wasters, the phone-wankers. I explained about the guys that were all going to see a mistress to get some kind of sexual kick that would get their rocks off. It made her think and realize that perhaps it wasn't the job she thought it was. At that point I realized how cynical I had become about the whole business and how I really just wanted some kind of normality. She thanked me for my time and I hoped she wouldn't call back.

I had been busy working so much over the past few months and had become very involved in the whole scene by doing videos and films as well as working as a dominatrix. I had a website jointly with another mistress and we would spend days at a time filming at the cottage. I would arrange for my subs to come and then we would shoot for the day. Adam, my best friend, and one of my subs would film the sessions and then edit them and then they would be put on the website. We had a number of members all over the world mostly from America, all watching me and another mistress with this so-called total power control. We would do cock ball torture, trample, strap-on, forced-bi, watersports, humiliation. I was starting to be recognized in the scene and was planning to go on a dom filming trip to Europe in a few months. Thousands of men were looking at my website and the movie site. Hundreds of them were downloading clips of me dominating men. Should I feel flattered or should I feel disgusted that these same men were probably having a sneaky wank over my pictures or videos in front of their pc while their wife had gone to bed early? Should I feel responsible for making grown men do disgusting things to each other by making them lick up their own cum or taking their virginity with my strap on or even worse forcing them to give oral sex to another man? Or should I realize that if I wasn't the instigator, they would be in some dirty men's toilet cottaging with some old pervert when all I was, was a conductor in a mixed up human orchestra that would direct them.

I remembered my favourite comedian a man that died a few years earlier. A man who was a revolutionary in his own right who didn't care about what other people thought about him and who had liberated a whole generation of people with his diverse humour and views on politics and sexuality. That man was Bills Hicks. I remembered the time when I had gone to see him live in concert in London when he talked about his love of oral sex and how he had the nickname "goatboy". He did a fantastic rendition of oral sex with a microphone that had me in stitches. I was sitting in the aisle with my eldest brother Sean and my mother. Then I remembered what he said. "my mother would be so proud of me". I laughed at the irony of my own situation. Yes I thought my mum would be really proud of me.

Perhaps it was time for me to move on. Perhaps it was time for me to stop and think about my life and how I was going to find a way of moving forwards. Lift myself out of this depression and feeling of hopelessness. Stop looking for answers by having destructive relationships with men, least of all those I would meet through work, who were likely to have far more issues than I ever had.

Rose Budworth Levine

I called Adam as he had spent the last few days trying to cheer me up. He always had a way of making me smile through adversity. We had discussed doing some different style of videos that wouldn't make me feel "too disgusted" and that would perhaps earn me some money. The latest craze was a new fetish called "Giantess". It was all videos of very large tall women who would trample and crush innocent victims and squash them with the power of their heels. The innocent victims were toys such as the matchbox cars my son Francis played with or vegetables and fruit and other inanimate objects. I decided I would go home that night and order myself some 8 inch heels and don myself in a latex catsuit that I had ordered a few days before. I would be 6 feet 5 in my new heels and tower over everything with my statuesque voluptuous figure that had commanded the attention of a many a mere mortal man. I had a pryor conversation with Dan one day a few months earlier and we had played a game of truth and dare. I asked him what his biggest sexual fantasy was and he said "to have interstellar sex with a latex clad spider woman." That was the reason I had ordered the suit. I wanted to wear it and have some photographs done of me in my photo gallery on the site in the small hope that Dan would one day go looking on my website again and feel regret at what he was missing. My revenge was always sweet although, be it in my head most of the time. That would be my new destiny, I said to myself, instead of trying to help what I thought was my lost soul. I would play the "giantess" and wear my new outfit with pride and squish innocent plastic men with my heels taking out my revenge on mankind. And in my head I would be thinking of Dan.

It was a freezing cold Monday morning. All my clients had cancelled for the day and I wasn't in the mood to work least of all get out of bed. My daughter did her usual trying to pretend she was sick because she didn't want to go to school but I managed after some confrontation to persuade her that she had to go. I mustered up the energy to get out of bed myself and go drop the children to school. The depression had taken a hold of me for weeks now, the migraines coming more frequently. Some mornings I was so bad I thought my head was going to either explode or implode on itself. It was always that constant pounding not to mention the extreme nausea and disorientation that went with migraine. How I hated those fucking headaches. Sometimes I felt it was god's way of punishing me for some misdemeanour I had done in a past life, and other times I just felt angry. Why did I have to have them all the time? It's bad enough having one every few months but I was getting them 2-3 times a week. I had been to the doctors and tried every cure possible. I had tried alternative remedies but the doctors said they were made worse by stress. How was I going to get rid of the stress in my life? I'd had it for months... I tried to objectify them by treating them as if they were someone else trying to get into my head. I'd woken up around 3am with a severe migraine a few months before. I texted Dan and I tried to explain how I felt when I was having one. He never had a headache despite drinking almost two bottles of wine every single day. The text read something like this: "that's right you fucking bastard you just keep on pounding away at my head with the same old tune. Mindless, tuneless drivel. Here we go! It's the lightshow now blah! blah! blah!

I got into my bed and pulled the covers up around my shoulders. I lay there quietly, still not wanting to move any part of my body, listening to the traffic noise passing my bedroom window. I thought about my life, about my regrets and I soon drifted off to into a dreamlike sleep dreaming about dying. I hoped I would wake up as someone else and wondered if I killed myself. Would I even know whether I was here anymore? Would there be that glorious light that everyone mentioned when they have a near death experience. Would I wake up in a new life as someone else and be startled by my own subconscious by remembering who I was or had been before? Would I just remain in a state of semi-consciousness for all eternity where I floated around aimlessly for the rest of my life, or would I wake up in heaven and become one with god and nature? Or would I end up in some miserable afterlife called hell? So many questions drifted in and out of my head as I lay there.

A few days later I still had the migraine. I'd been spending the last few days drifting in and out of reality trying to look after the children with this pounding headache that just wouldn't go. It was a

INTIMATE ENCOUNTERS

Tuesday evening and Francis was due to go to his regular Tae kwon do lesson but needed some help with his homework. I could hardly stand without feeling dizzy and I was trying to cook dinner for the children. I realized the dog didn't have any food so I called my daughter and asked her to finish off cooking and jumped in the car and drove to the pet store. I felt like I was in this altered state of consciousness, how I managed to drive the car and get home I am not sure. Most people would have migraines and have to retire to their beds for a few hours. I'd have recurrent migraines and still managed to work.

I woke up the next morning feeling desperate. How could I manage to get through the next few weeks? Christmas was coming in a couple of weeks and I hadn't even thought about buying presents or cards. I wanted to run; I wanted to be as far away from myself as possible. That was the key, I wanted to run away from me. I'd spent so much time living a constant 'out of body experience' with the headaches I almost convinced myself I could physically detach myself. I believed I was starting to go insane. I tried to call Dan that morning; I didn't dare to speak to him and left a message with a member of staff asking him to call me back. I knew that we were finished I didn't even want to have a relationship with him anymore; in fact I didn't even like him much the way he'd been acting the past few weeks. In my mind, I just wanted him to come and see me and say something that would snap me out of this miserable dark hole. I felt like I was drowning at the bottom of a Well and couldn't breath. He had talked about feeling suicidal himself so I thought he understood but he talked about lots of things and did little. I wanted someone to rescue me and pull me out. I imagined that he was just laughing at me thinking I was some crazy schizophrenic woman that was stalking him. The reality was, I had only phoned him on my most desperate days usually once every week or two. I had no other way of contacting him, I didn't know where he lived and he had told me he'd lost his mobile phone and wasn't going to get another one. How stupid did he think I was to believe he wouldn't have a phone when his father was about to die and may need to call him at any time. However I was the one that was dying I was the one that didn't feel like I had the strength or inclination to hold out until the New Year. I wasn't even sure if I saw him whether it would make any difference to the way I was feeling. Chances were, that I was so low I would have another relapse in a couple of days and want to kill myself again.

How I despised him for his selfishness and arrogance. This was a man that had looked up to me and told me that he would always be a friend to me no matter what. This was a man that couldn't see anything, couldn't see that I was sick. If I have had a physical illness that he could see, would he have even bothered to call me then, probably not? You see for Dan it was all about him, he thought me wanting to kill myself was because of him it wasn't at all it was because I just had too much on.

INTIMATE ENCOUNTERS

9 - THE DEAD SEA

I felt the best thing I could do under the circumstances was to run, only this time it would be a "controlled" run with my children. Two weeks away on holiday just before Christmas with my children. Egypt seemed like a good place to go. I texted Dan and said we were finished and jumped on a plane a few days later. We had a glorious few weeks away. My head still hurt, the pain still there but it gave me a few weeks to forget all my troubles, me debt, my obsession with Dan, my headaches, the problems I was having with the 'Mistress Vile' and then I would return home refreshed and recharged. It gave me time to find myself again, find out who Rose was, I wasn't the Dom on holiday I was a princess. I spent the holiday just relaxing for the first time in over two years. The constant work and debts meant I never had more than a moment to sit down so I just enjoyed the glorious weather the hot sun and the sea. It reminded me of my time years ago when I was young and beautiful and had backpacked, when I was single had no responsibility, when I was innocent when I was free and when I was happy. I had taken the children snorkeling and darks thoughts had surfaced again so I wrote a poem while I was away.

As I lie in my bed I drift and fly
Illusions of grandeur fill my eyes
My head hurts so much I want to shout
A bashful of tears seems the only way out

Rose Budworth Levine

Broken promises and shattered dreams
Dreaming of monsters and squashing ice creams

Take me down to the Red sea
I want to clear my head and be free
Take me down to the Red sea
I want to clear my head and be free

With weightlessness comes clarity
At one with nature my mind set free
I look in the eyes of the ones I created
Hopes of forgiveness and not hatred
Happiness comes to us just fleetingly
Its given in moments of pure ecstasy

Take me down to the Red sea
The "I don't want to be dead" sea
Take me down to the Red sea
The "I don't want to be dead" sea

As I drift and dream in this open space
For once in my life I have found my place
I find myself almost effortlessly
Feeling the joy of just being me
The fish smile back they know who I am
I can stay here forever in this wonderland

Bring me back up from the Red Sea
And free me from this insanity
Bring me back up from the Red Sea
And free me from this insanity

Back home I am faced with reality

INTIMATE ENCOUNTERS

A pile of letters staring back at me
My eyes fill up with a hundred tears
Its all monsters and demons and same old fears
Dear god I am on bended knee
Please give me the strength to just be

Don't take me back to the Red Sea
I am trying so hard not to be dead you see
Don't take me back to the Red sea
I am trying so hard not to be dead you see

My suntan fading as fast as my dreams
Back to the monsters and squishing ice creams
I look in the mirror it stares back at me
I don't have the strength anymore to be me
Life just an illusion a difficult game
Its hard to play it when your going insane

Throw my ashes back in the Dead Sea
Because now I am nothing but Dead you see
Throw my ashes back in the Dead Sea
Because now I am nothing but Dead you See

So I am here again on bending knee
Hope those I left behind will forgive me
I look down below and admire the bubbles
Float up and disperse along with my troubles
No one cares here about my insanity
I'll stay here forever and be whatever I wanna be

Now I can dream of the Red Sea
The "I don't want to be dead sea
Now I can dream of the Red Sea

Rose Budworth Levine

Because now my soul and mind is set free

I came home feeling somewhat better and more relaxed but I came back down to earth with a bump.

It was Christmas Eve and there were a pile of debts waiting for me on the hall table. I didn't dare open them. Dan had finally sent me a text saying he would contact me on Christmas day. As was always the case, his limits on time and space weren't quite the same as everyone else and I received a call on Boxing Day. I wasn't quite sure why he had phoned me; probably the Christmas spirit had got the better of him. We talked on the phone and he explained that he didn't want any headache, and that he had been freaked-out by the whole thing of me being sick and needing him, and couldn't cope. Then in the next breath he was asking me if he could come and see me on his day off. He always confused me for some reason, or maybe it was just the headaches that were confusing me? Maybe it was just the madness from the constant pain I had every day that was deluding me? Either way I wanted to see him. Of course Thursday came and went and I got a call to say he couldn't come over but would be there Friday. Friday came. He texted me to say he had a problem at home and was going to be kicked out of his place. As always, I offered to help and sent him a few texts to say if he needed anything I was there for him. He texted me back to say thank you and said he would call the next day.

INTIMATE ENCOUNTERS

When I finally managed to get on the PC on my return, I checked my emails and site and while I was away Shirley had emailed my subs and had finished doing nearly 300 films in a month, almost to the point of obsession. She had got her husband to be in the films and done the most outrageous videos, severe forced bi-fucking and needle-play. Coming from a woman that was phobic about needles this seems a little worrying. All of the films she had done had been filmed in the boys bedroom and she had taken turns to let total strangers baby-sit the boys while she was busy fucking some guy upstairs up the arse at the same time. I have always kept my private business away from my children and this was something she was doing in front of children that had little understanding and should never have been exposed to it.

I wanted out, so I told her I wanted to build my own site and we would run the two along side and split the money and as she had enough content herself. She threatened to sue me if I did anything with the site and said I was not to take one penny out of the bank account. I wanted to phone the police and tell them this woman was a complete monster but I was scared she would retaliate and then my whole world would be turned upside down. My daughter confronted me one day and said she knew I was a dominatrix because Shirley had left something on the PC and she had overheard a conversation. She had been wondering for some time. I nicknamed her Mistress Vile. I was gutted that what I had fought so long to hide from my daughter had been found out with a small mistake.

I cried and tried to explain myself and my daughter said to me. "You know what mum I don't care what you do. I know you're not a prostitute, so long as I don't know the details I am fine. I love you you're my mum". I managed to rebuild my site working day and night so I could give Mistress Vile the site back in her name. I had migraines every single day. Then the day I was due to hand it back over I received an email. I had forgotten that she had access to my email account once when I had to check a booking for a client and still had the password. She had been reading my private emails for months. There was an email, which my new web designer wrote in confidence saying that she was a nasty piece of work and that I was well rid of her which she quoted. He email said that she had withdrawn what she thought was owed to her and to stick the website up my arse. She withdrew three and a half grand from the bank and left me with 1,500 for 6 months of work. 14 hours of video footage down the drain and months rebuilding my site again for nothing.

After that she slipped into a real case of what I can only describe on the scene as dominatrix toxemia. It's where a dominatrix believes her own hype. Often it stems from lack of confidence whereby they feel the only way they can feel worthy is to have these slaves who pander to their every wishes and tell them what a goddess they are. I could never suffer from Dom toxemia, I only had to look in the mirror and see my wrinkles and roots showing through or my cellulite. And besides I didn't believe most of the shit these guys said anyway. It was just their dicks talking. Once they had come, thoughts of "I love my mistress and I will do anything for you", went right out the window. But Shirley was different she wanted to be something; she had been created by her husband and had to find her own niche. She was watching my website all the time. Everything I did she copied and tried to do better. She tried to email all my slaves and get them to go and become film slaves for her. Those of them that were stupid enough to go and see her ended up on a downward spiral of BDSM and had to be branded and collared to be her slaves. She became house dominatrix at a number of clubs and had visions of becoming a channel four presenter. She started to do extreme needle play having had no experience or training in anatomy. I had a call one day from a friend to say that she was blackmailing slaves and that one of her clients had died. I couldn't believe that this woman had been my friend. Her husband became her cuckold and she took on a string of lovers and he delighted at being cleanup boy but, cleaning up all the spunk after she had been fucked, when all the time I knew that the driving force behind her domination was insecurity and sheer hatred of her own husband. With any kind of job comes responsibility and this woman was a lose cannon.

It was New Years Eve and I was dreading it. I had already asked Dan if he would take me out for the evening and break the cycle of staying in and having a bad new year for the past five. As I expected he had already arranged something long before. I knew where I stood on his list of priorities, even as a friend let alone a lover; I didn't stand a chance of ever being part of his life. Good old Adam had arranged to come up for the evening so I wouldn't be alone. I got a call from Betty one of the subs I had filmed with in the past. He was a chemistry teacher who had a penchant for spanking and bottom worship. I decided in my wisdom to invite him up for New Years Eve too. After all Adam and me weren't going to be doing much. Probably a few worship foot videos to pass the time and take my mind off my problems.

It was my daughters birthday a day or so later. She had tried to reconcile her differences with her father and he had offered a vacant house for her to have her birthday and New Year celebration. She had promised me that she would call either her father or me if there was any problem. Both of us were only a few minutes away in the car. I was at the cottage having just finished filming some squish food videos and Betty was busying herself upstairs in preparation for a New Year spanking. I received a call from her father to say there had been a gas leak at the house and everyone had been evacuated and the police had turned up. I jumped in the car and got Adam to drive me there. When I arrived I found a house with my daughter completely drunk and the whole place had been trashed. There were gaping holes in the walls where kids had taken it upon themselves to kick the plasterwork in; there was piss and vomit all over the house. Cigarettes stubbed out on new flooring just laid. The whole house was a mess. A bunch of kids gone crazy on alcohol and been skating in the living room and trashed everything. Even the food in the fridge had been used and the whole place had been turned into a bombsite within a few hours.

Her father stood there so disappointed. She had lashed out at him and accidentally smashed his face in the door and then laughed at him because of her drunkenness. I took her home and went to say goodbye to Betty and see in the New Year albeit for an hour. It had to be the most surreal messed up New Year I have had. Most of my recent past New Years had been crap but this one had really taken the biscuit. I decided next year had to be better. I didn't want to be spending my new year with a TV maid nor worrying about whether my daughter was going to kill herself.

The following week I received a call from one of my friends Julie saying that her best friend Donna who I knew a little had committed suicide and I was asked to go to the funeral. Her ex husband has insisted on taking the children over Christmas, piled with debts and just having come out of a destructive relationship similar to the one I was in with Dan I went to the funeral feeling very apprehensive hoping I wouldn't break down. Her sons played with my own son at school and she was a good mother. No one had any idea she had felt suicidal not even her best friend. But Donna had made a call to her the day before and she was busy. They found her with all the boys

Rose Budworth Levine

Christmas presents wrapped up and a pile of pills and booze dead in her house. She was a nurse so she knew what she was doing. A note to her boys saying she loved them that was that. Everyone at the funeral was angry and upset at her for leaving her boys behind. They played some beautiful music she liked, everyone said their bit. Tears streamed down my face, I just felt like I was going to my own funeral. That's how I had been feeling for months. That's what would happen if had committed suicide, no sympathy just anger and hurt from all the family and not understanding that when you reach the bottom sometimes its just so hard to pull yourself back out. I had done it on many occasions, pulled myself back. It was usually the fear of not doing the job properly, or being riddled with guilt for life for wanting to get out. There would always be something that would pick me up off the floor and it would always be myself.

It was late January, after a month on HRT which had only served to make my migraines worse I ended up in casualty. My head hurt so much I didn't care whether I lived or died at that point I just wanted fixing, even the doctor in casualty commented on how impossible it would be for anyone to cope with migraines 24 hours a day for 3 months. I was finally going to see a neurologist who would help me to get better but it didn't feel like anything was getting better. I had started to see Dan again, he had spent Christmas and New Year getting "pissed up" then made a new years resolution to come off the drink and go back to college. I even gave him acupuncture and he was off the booze for a week. But then Dan always made promises he couldn't keep like he would promise to call. The only person he ever really let down was himself. I wanted out again, the bills were piling up partly my own fault for booking a holiday I could hardly afford, partly for not being able to work for over 6 weeks, partly for not having any domination work for a while. I was juggling credit card bills by the dozen and my head was pounding every single minute of the day. Dan knew I was having a bad week and I had warned him I might need to call him for help. He always knew what that meant and said if you need me I will be there anytime you want day or night. He had a habit of switching his phone off for days but he had been much better these past few months. It was Monday morning and I had planned it all. I wrote all the letters and decided to pack up the whole dungeon. I didn't want my family knowing what I had been up to for the past few years so I knew if I "opted out" I needed a plan.

I had written a note to Adam and one to my mum and dad, one to my children and one to Dan. I had been seeing a slave by the name of 'H', he had become a very good friend, coming over regularly and helping me at the cottage, filming, his uncle had recently died and been found in the woods and he had remained so calm. I knew if anything was going to happen to me he would. This was the person that would be able to cope with everything and it seemed like he liked me and

Rose Budworth Levine

I trusted him. So I packed everything up over a whole week. I packed everything up in a rather organized fashion in between sobbing. I thought if I was going to take my life then I could stupidly get someone to come and empty the cottage before the police would even have a chance to find out what had happened. It took me 3 days in all to pack everything up and I arranged for my children to stay with their father on the Friday night and booked into a hotel near Birmingham so that I could carry out my plan. I wanted someone to rescue me, I didn't really want to go but I was desperate didn't know any other way out of this hole I was in. I tried to call slave H a couple of times that week but he didn't answer his phone, so finally I called Dan. It was the Friday morning. didn't get a reply so I sent him a text saying I was feeling really wobbly and would it be ok if I came over that evening just for ten minutes after work. The next thing I got a call from his work. I was in the car with the children and he seemed to be in a state of panic, concerned that I was already on my way over in the car. I explained that I wasn't and that I was just feeling really dreadful and wanted just a bit of his time after work. He said "i'm sorry I can't do it, I am afraid I will be too tired after work".

I went home that evening, with a large bottle of paracetamol in my handbag. I dropped the children at their father's house. I never did go to the hotel. I went on the Internet and looked up 'Suicide' on the internet. I read somewhere that suicide by paracetamol and alcohol overdose is one of the most excruciatingly painful ways to die and there is not guarantee that you will die but you can be sure of permanent liver damage. I thought to myself why the hell am I doing this when someone I thought cared has no concern for me whatsoever. I cried for about 36 hours. Francis called me the next day saying "please can we come home Mum as we miss you so much. I picked them up and told them I had had a migraine which is why my eyes where puffed up. I am not sure that they believed me, and I sent a text to Dan the next day explaining that I would never see him again.

10 - MR MARRIED AND MISUNDERSTOOD

They say "never go out with someone on the rebound", its so true! I always had many different slaves coming and going from the dungeon. There was my longest-term friend Adam who stayed at the weekends, he had become a friend of the family. Although no one knew he was a submissive they just thought he was a mate. He was always there for me whenever I needed picking up or was in the shit. Everyone wanted some part of me in oneway or another. I was single and after finishing with Dan there was no exception.

One of my so-called slaves had been coming for some time about a year I guess. His name was Jamie, and I had nicknamed him slave. He was very level headed and was the person I had written my suicide note to, asking to organize everything when I had gone. The letter had explained how to get rid of all the dungeon furniture and clear up the evidence. One of his uncles had died a few months earlier and he had been so matter of fact about it and very calm. I knew he would be the only one that would be able to sort things out for me. He had originally come for a session but then helped out in the dungeon doing films etc. I remember when I first set eyes on him, thinking how handsome he was so I gave him a nickname which would reflect that. But he was married and I never really thought much about until a few weeks after things had finished between me and Dan. I had just got rid of Mistress

INTIMATE ENCOUNTERS

Vile and had been reading a book called "Bad Boys – why we love them" about women who choose destructive relationships. I realized in all my relationships with men in the past I had played second best. I was second to my first boyfriend with all his other girlfriends, second to my ex husband with all his family, and second to my ex and his drugs and cheating. Now I had been second to Dan and the alcohol. I was repeating the same old pattern again and again. I least I was realizing something. Eureka I thought the penny has finally dropped!

Jamie was different for all the rest, he reminded me of my brother Sean in many ways. It was the first time I had made a friendship with a man and not jumped into bed, although I had many male friends far more than I had women. But it was much more than that; I was extremely attracted to him. We had a long meaningful chat about how he understood and would be there for me to help me though as a friend, and then I laughed and said "you know, perhaps I just should forget about relationships and just have the odd shag now and then" He replied" well if you ever need a shag". The next minute I was on his lap kissing him and we were making love in bed together. We had the most amazing sex I had had in a very long time. My legs were shaking. I told him after when he explained how he never made love to his wife and how they hadn't had sex for months. I just laughed and said "well you know what I am a big girl you don't need to tell me that to get in my knickers" If we are going to have a relationship even just sex I want you to be completely honest with me always and he promised that he would always.

We had been seeing each other for a couple of weeks when just after making love one day he said to me "you do realize I am falling madly in love with you and that I will leave my wife for you" I think I let my guard down then. Or maybe I didn't have any guards to let down. The next few months I started to feel better, to feel good about myself again. I started to make plans about the future; I wanted to have a new life, one that would include Jamie. Jamie was happy with me doing the domination, in fact he got excited at me doing some of it, and he even joined in on the filming and the sessions. He started to switch and I even let him dominate me a few times which was fun. I even started to get rid of some of the baggage I had been carrying around for years by losing weight. I lost nearly 3 1/2 stone during that year. I felt happy most of the time. We spend a year having a wonderful time enjoying each others company meeting up when he could get away from his wife and playing.

That was until one day when I realized he might not be around for much longer. The day he found out he had cancer. I cried so many tears feeling helpless because I wanted to help him. All I could do is just listen; I couldn't even go see him in hospital. Then I started to torture myself emotionally thinking about what would happen if he didn't come through. I wouldn't even be able to go to the funeral. Each day we saw each other the

INTIMATE ENCOUNTERS

tension grew over his marriage. I thought he would definitely leave when he found out he had cancer. Especially as I had been the one who had pointed it out to him. His wife was too busy to even notice he had this horrible slow growing growth on his head that had got bigger during the year. It was a difficult time in every way, my daughter had started to smoke pot and hang around with the wrong crowd. I don't know what was worse, her smoking spliffs or cutting herself as she had done a couple of years before.

During our relationship we spent two nights away during that time. Once when it was my birthday, he took me to a hotel for the evening. He got drunk and I got sick, which was just funny really. The second was his birthday and I had arranged to see a woman who specialized in Tantric sex. I wanted to have a birthday he would remember and one that I could enjoy too. It was a day that would connect us deeply and take me away from my everyday problems, paying bills, looking after the kids, the fact that he was there with her and not with me one that would help him forget that he had cancer. That day was going to be all about us.

It was a strange day. I had spoken to her on the phone a few times and wasn't quite sure what to expect. We had planned to stay the whole day then spend the night in Bath going to a restaurant. She was the most beautiful angelic looking woman with the innocence of a child. Although she was nearly fifty she had the body of a young woman. Her skin was fresh and clear, long blonde hair without makeup. We had an introductory chat about what I expected. I remember her saying on the phone how she could work magic in her own way. Minouska talked to Jamie about his life, his wife and his cancer. Told him he should leave her and be true to himself otherwise he would end up being sick and unhappy. She explained how we both had this very rare connection that should be nurtured. I think at one point he thought it was a set up. I put my head down thinking "oh my god, she's supposed to be helping me and here she is telling my boyfriend how he is in denial and should leave his wife." When we eventually started the day, the lighting was soft, music was gentle and candles flicked over our bodies as we stroked touched and she guided us on this spiritual sexual journey. There wasn't much Jamie hadn't already touched on before we met her, it was just an affirmation of where our relationship was and I went out of there on cloud nine feeling calm, rejuvenated and at one with myself and him.

But then the big downer, as we walked hand in hand to the car, it was dark by now. Jamie opened the car door to check his phone. We were greeted by an angry call from his wife. Something about some bill he hadn't paid and why he hadn't answered the phone all day. I can't quite remember, nor did I care. I never smoked when he was around because of his cancer. Often I would go for the whole day. I walked off into the dark of the night, found myself sitting on the bench lighting up a cigarette. He called me about twenty minutes later to ask me where I was. I walked back to the car and we drove back to the hotel, I think I was crying. I guess I would always feel like that while he was still married. I was pissed and angry that she had spoiled our day.

The following day after a lovely meal and a long drive back home, I talked about my plans for the future. How I wanted to become a sex therapist, using my experience as a dominatrix and perhaps combining it with the Tantra we had learnt the day before. I planned to spend the next couple of years training to be a counselor. We had talked on many occasions about setting up a business together, with his interests in martial arts and mine in therapy; I could start to do something positive again. I wanted to do something that would not make me feel as demeaning as the domination did which was now becoming soul destroying as all I was doing was using it to pay off my huge debts.

Halfway through the journey I realized he had either called her on route at the service station, or changed plans and wanted to get back early. My car was parked near his hometown instead of mine and it meant I had to go collect my car first to get back home. He said he was worried that if he dropped me near my car she might see me while she was on the school run. I went into panic mode, one of many, and asked him to drop me miles from my car in the middle of town, I was crying. He said he didn't want to just leave me but I just felt I had just been dumped. We had just been away for an amazing couple of days and now he couldn't wait to get rid of me. He managed to persuade me to get back into the car and drove me back to mine. It was a couple of days before we spoke again. Everything spoilt as usual until the next time we would make love have a nice day together and then she would come back into the conversation again one way or another. If it wasn't him always having to rush back home to look after the kids, he would be complaining to me how she didn't understand him, how he had all their in-laws living with him. How he was just there paying all the bills. I found the whole thing very soul destroying and my self-esteem was starting to sink.

I started to feel really bad about myself wondering why he wouldn't leave her. I knew Christmas was coming up in a few months and the last thing I wanted to do was spend it in England thinking about playing happy families with his wife. Although he kept promising to leave, he had made it very clear he had no immediate plans and I would just have to wait, So as usual, my impulsiveness and stupidity got the better of me and I booked a holiday for me and the kids to go away at Christmas and new year to Thailand.

In hindsight it was the last thing I could afford to do but being optimistic I thought I'd be able to sell the property, I had just bought, to do up in time. Work was picking up so why not spoil myself at least I wouldn't be thinking about him. But then they booked his operation while I was due to be away. That really bothered me wondering what might happen to him, would he come round because he was asthmatic?

It was a month or so before Christmas when I got a call from my brother Sean in the states. His wife who had been depressed during her pregnancy had given birth early and had a breakdown and been committed in hospital. He was beside himself. I immediately booked a flight, arranged for my parents to look after the children and within a week I was on the plane. I arrived still jetlagged and looked after my nephew for the next ten days. His wife had now been released but was very sick. She wanted to be rid of the baby the easiest way possible by adopting him out. I guess I realized how sick she was when she ran naked in the flat one night kneeling on the floor begging Sean to get rid of him and started to cut wrists with a knife saying "if you love me you will get rid of the baby". I think she was probably schizophrenic triggered off by the pregnancy. Sean couldn't cope, he was working full-time as a teacher and studying and the baby had been looked after various different "mummies" while he managed his schedule. I told Sean how my situation was at home and that I was working as a dominatrix and he wasn't surprised. It was a relief to tell someone in the family and stop living a lie. He said well "you and me are quite similar we are fucked up when it comes to sex and relationships". Look at me" he said "Married twice before. The last marriage I had I disappeared off to Thailand for a month after my wife had to terminate our baby due to ill health which broke my marriage down" I shagged everything in site. "I have wanted a child all my life, now I have one I don't have a wife that can look after him". I suggested I take the baby home with me and I would look after him until he was able to cope, and that my mum would help when I was at work during the day. The baby was sent off to spend a few weeks with another member of the family while we were organizing his passports and paperwork. I knew I would need a holiday now I had committed myself, so off I flew to Thailand.

I never thought about the consequences, my motherly instinct just took over, I never thought about how I wouldn't be able to work as much and get into even more debt, how my house would not get finished, how my health might eventually end up suffering, or how I would have weeks of sleepless nights looking after a screaming baby that would end up thinking of me as his own mummy.

Thailand was amazing, the most beautiful people I have met spiritually. There is a lot to be said for Buddhism. We stayed in a very quiet hotel near Kao Lak. It wasn't until we arrived I realized that it was one of the hotels and resorts that had been completely wiped out by the tsunami two Christmases before. The children fell in love with it. We talked about how materialistic everything was back home. My children are free spirits they have been bought up to think as individuals and to have their own opinions. We talked about moving there about selling everything up and making a new start. They were happy to see their mum smiling again. The warmth of the sun on my face,

INTIMATE ENCOUNTERS

the freedom from everyday debts and worries drained from my face each day that I stayed. We met a charismatic tour guide called Emma who shared the same birthday and name as my own daughter. Emma had nearly lost her life at 'Phi Phi Island' and had lost her boyfriend. She spent weeks searching for him.

We met many people like Emma and found the whole experience very humbling. We invited her to come with us at New Year to 'Krabi'. Myself and the kids went to a rave party in the middle of a rubber wood forest while she stayed with her friends. She said it wasn't her thing. We joined up the next morning and she took us to a beautiful mangrove swamp where we swam and had breakfast with the locals. How idyllic it would be to come out here and live. My friend Pasquale was also in Thailand planning to set up a retreat and wanted me to move out there too. I was torn between staying at home and working things out with the boyfriend and taking a chance on a new life away from all the stress I had had for the past few years. My mind wandered as usual, I was daydreaming, we ate breakfast and I was happy but tired and we had a long way to drive back. We all piled into the car and then BANG I had been in such a dream like state and busy making sure I didn't run anyone over coming out of the car park that I failed to notice a tree behind me in the shape of a V. You couldn't see it out of the rear mirror and the stump had taken the back end off the brand new hire car. That was New Year's Day.

I drove back with the boot tied up; exhaust hanging off, crying most of the way and wondering whether this was how the rest of my year would pan out.

I got home and the following week I received an email. My websites had all gone. The web host had gone bust. I had spent a year rebuilding them after the episode with Mistress Vile and now I had to start again. I was ready to jack it all in there and then but I couldn't, I had so much debt to pay off. I was juggling credit card bills every month and no one else was going to pay my mortgage payments. So I started all over again rebuilding my site, putting my members site back up again and just did everything day by day until I couldn't do anymore. Some days I struggled.

A mutual friend called to say they heard that I had received a call from a mutual friend to say Shirley's husband had got his inheritance and he had got 4.2 million and that she had kicked him out and filed for divorce. She had herself a nice boyfriend and was flaunting the fact that she was as happy as a pig in shit. I thought to myself considering life and Karma and all things that were going on in own life, that life just didn't seem very fair lately. It was one of those "princess and the pea" days as I like to think of them. I hardly tell anyone but I have a pain condition called 'Fibiromyalgia' along with a slipped disc that flares up from time to time. I have struggled for many years with it since the birth of my son. Most days I manage but occasionally it just hurts. It's the kind of pain where you feel like you have had two rounds with Mike Tyson in the ring. If anyone were to poke or prod me or even touch me I would winch. The children were kind of used to it. I wouldn't complain to them just say "give me a cuddle another time" or something along those lines. Often it was worse if I hadn't slept well the night before and being an insomniac it didn't really help matters much. I dream frequently having done so since I was a child and frequently I talk in my sleep, more so when I am under stress

As a child my mother used to stand outside my bedroom door sometimes trying to have conversations with me while I was asleep. I had a dream the night before about both my ex husbands, they were both poking and prodding me and in my side, punching me while no one was looking. As I was being beaten, each one sniggering while the other one was punching me. It was 5 am and the baby had woken up so I had to go make him a bottle. . When I got up I could hardly get myself down the stairs I felt like I had been beaten up. Perhaps there was a connection, maybe I was beating myself up and letting everyone else beat me up some more, and that's why I had the pain.

I guess I always knew that domination was always about the submissive and in a way it was I that was the submissive, always working for them, it was really no different from doing any other nine to five job. It really hit home that I wanted to pack up doing it professionally when I had arranged to do a professional video for a promotional company. Obviously they were out for their pound of flesh. The guy that filmed was loaded and had enough money to go on luxury holidays every year with his wife who was an ex Dom. We had made arrangements to do a two day shoot. I organized for my best subs and slaves to be in the film, I even roped in the boyfriend. We all had to sign model release forms and I would have loved to have seen the look on his wife's face if she had gone into her local sex shop and found a video of her husband being dominated. That would have certainly gotten him into the divorce courts if nothing else.

All the subs turned up on the Thursday, and I wasn't really in the mood to be playing the role of mistress having had a migraine all week. I guess I should give a little background into perhaps why I might have had a migraine. You see my stress levels were always a bit high, to say the least. Most people would find one job stressful i.e. looking after two children is enough but me well I just like to take on the world.

My daughter Emma had decided in her wisdom the week before that she never wanted to go to school again, not the best of good timing when you only have 9 weeks to go until the end of school and your GCSE's to finish. I had just returned a couple of months earlier from the states having promised to be "auntie mum" and I was up to my eyeballs in babysitting my 4 month old brothers Sean's baby, whose wife had abandoned him. I'd had six weeks of sleepless nights up bottle feeding every couple of hours. I was domming

INTIMATE ENCOUNTERS

during the day, looking after a new baby, looking after the kids, running my therapy business, collecting the rent from my properties and trying to sell my house, paying off huge credit card bills and basically running around like a blue arsed fly, so doing a debut domination movie with a bunch of needy subs that wanted all my attention wasn't probably a very good idea.

So, back to Thursday night. I'd asked Jamie to come over and we had planned to spend a nice romantic evening on our own after filming all day. The last thing I wanted was to spend it with a load of subs. I'd arranged for my father to come up with my stepmother to look after the baby, since I had told the family I was on a course for a couple of days. I couldn't very well tell them I was going on a video making guys do forced Bi and torturing their cocks.

Two of my subs hadn't shown up for the shoot. One of them had bottled it because of the model release form, even though he wore a mask, and the other slave was worried about his wife seeing him on video. So at the last minute I had arranged for a TV friend to come over and help out. I knew it would be really stressful dreaming up storylines for the film and I was under pressure to churn out 10 hours of video over two days. The first day went fine and Jamie and I had booked to go to a Thai restaurant in town. Simon my TV friend wanted to come out with us and so did the delightful 'Betty'. I wasn't really in the mood to spend my 1-year anniversary with them but we all went out together anyway.

Rose Budworth Levine

We enjoyed the meal, it was a Thai restaurant, and it reminded me how I wished I were back in Thailand away from all the pressure. How life was so simple there. How my children had wanted me to pack everything up and go and move there with them but I had decided to stay because I wanted to make things work out with my married boyfriend. We got a few strange glances from some of the other people in the restaurant as Betty still had nail polish from the film shoot earlier. We were talking about transvestites, domination and general BDSM.

Earlier that evening my so-called romantic plans were obviously thrown out of the window, with Jamie I had sneaked off upstairs into the dungeon room. We always had a great sex life but it was the first time that he couldn't get excited. I think the penny had finally dropped. He had tears in his eyes and it was the first time in ages that he had started to resonate with me again. He said, "Rose, everyone wants a bit of you. And I don't feel happy with you doing the domination anymore professionally". "Thank god for that! I finally thought". I'd been trying to get out of it, all this business all the time, but because we both enjoyed playing the roles, since part of him got at excited at me being the "dominatrix".

He went back home to his wife and I stayed with Simon and Betty. Cumalot came over pissed up, wanting a prostitute as he was staying at the local hotel. I was in my pyjamas worn out from the day ready to go to bed I told him to go home and get some sleep for the next day. I slept with

INTIMATE ENCOUNTERS

Simon in the spare room trying quietly not to snore. Cumalot was still busy chatting downstairs with Betty. I received a text the next day saying he couldn't show up for the shoot. He had got his rocks off the night before and blood had came out which meant he needed to go see a doctor. I was so glad when those two days were over.

11- THE EPIPHANY

So a few weeks later, everything had started to crash around me. I was just too overloaded. I felt like a pack of cards stacked up waiting to fall. It was now five months that I had been looking after my nephew; he was teething and crying often. The house I had bought, with all my hopes and dreams for a future with my boyfriend, and pay off my debts with, had not sold. I had bought a new kitchen a couple of months ago and needed to have it fitted so I had gone back to my old pattern of forgiving my ex husband for not paying maintenance and arranged for him to fit my kitchen instead of paying me for the kids. I laughed when my kitchen arrived, remembering how I had bought it from a local kitchen company and how the owner who had a girlfriend had tried to chat me up. I laughed how I'd ended up telling him I was a dominatrix and he had come for a session and because I couldn't afford to get it fitted he had kept it in his showroom for months scared that his girlfriend might find out he had been to see me. Men were such simple creatures I thought, you could play with them any way you wanted. I was good at playing the game but that's all it was, a big bloody game. My house was a tip, covered in brick dust, it was half term for school, I couldn't work and I had to find two grand by the end of the month to pay the mortgages alone. My migraines were back, my coil that had been fitted to stop my periods needed changing and I had been 'on' for eight days.

INTIMATE ENCOUNTERS

I guess it all came crashing down the day I went surfing on the web. Bert, the guy that had shot the video with always liked to come across as "Mister nice guy". I had told him about a website I put some films on. He had started to make money for himself. As a favour he offered to send up some of my films to them. I should have done it myself by I had so much on. He explained that it was very complicated and that it would be easier if he did it for me. I should have known he was going to rip me off when my member's sites he built was only bringing in 30 per month and my own. One I did myself was netting about 250. But in hindsight I didn't. So I was surfing the net and found a clip on the net. It was a film about face sitting and referred to a specific artist that did cartoon pictures of face sitting. What I had done in the video is bought the character to life. It had taken months of planning. Even with the domination I had tried to hard to do my best. There was no mention of my mistress name just a reference to the guy in the clip and the description said "Namio loves a little face smothering now and then – actually he loves it all the fucking time! He can't get enough of his big fat neighbour coming over and sitting on his face with her dirty panties and even dirtier smelly Cunt! Nothing gets him off more than breathing in some smelly puss!" All the rest of the clips didn't even refer to me, even though I now had a reputation as a well known international dominatrix.

There I was on the floor, sobbing uncontrollable and that's exactly how I felt, some fat cow, except that everyone was sitting, or should I say, shitting on me. He didn't even have permission to put those on my own site. I emailed him and said I may not be a beauty queen but I am a dominatrix not some fat tart with a stinking puss, when half of the women on your site are working as prostitutes. And then I thought about it for a while and thought, actually, I am no better than them. I had been receiving texts all week from different subs saying, "Please mistress will you use your big strap-on on me. Will you smother me until I pass out and then piss on me to wake me up, Mistress I love you but let me lick the spunk off your boots, I am a TV that loves to be "forced" to suck cocks while being dressed as a slut. And even I will do anything for you mistress even eat your shit! And that was pretty normal. It all made me laugh! Forced? My arse! Submissives weren't forced to do anything that wasn't on their list of wishes. They only let mistresses do things to them that they wanted done. It was all about them. As for shit, I was letting everyone shit on me because I was allowing it.

Before that realization of course I was still crying about the episode with the webguy. I had a migraine, the dog had been tied up outside for a couple of days while the kitchen was being knocked through and had been barking for a few days. We lived next door to a neighbour married with four children; two of his sons were gay. He was an angry man. We had been good neighbours for years we would always look after each other's animals when we went on holiday, his wife would pop in for a coffee and we would even drop cakes and food off to each other when we had been cooking. We had fallen out over a brick wall, laughable really. It was my boundary wall and his tree was growing out of it. I was up to my eyeballs in debt and couldn't afford to get the wall rebuilt. My best friend had come round to help me sort out the attic, I had a habit of hoarding shit and not letting go and I had warned him not to put anything over the wall and to wait till the morning. I found him in the garden laying on the floor the wall had collapsed with him the dog licking him.

So this bloody wall needed rebuilding now. I spoke to the neighbour who agreed to give me hundred quid towards the cost of building it. Weeks passed and I hadn't got around to getting it fixed but he never mentioned anything. I had taken the wall down and had all the old bricks cleaned up ready to build. Then one day I was out in the garden and he had taken all the bricks and built his own wall. So when I confronted him on the phone he was very angry. I put a very polite note through the door saying it was a shame he hadn't mentioned it before and how it would be a shame not to discuss it. They never spoke to me again. In fact neither did his wife nor his kids. They wouldn't even look at me or my own children from that day forward, or my children that they happily played with in the garden a few months before.

That was until a few months later when I had bought the house next door to them, to repay my debts. His thoughts were obviously that I was absolutely loaded so I swallowed my pride and explained to him why I was buying the house and how upset I had been that they hadn't spoken to me for two years over a bloody brick wall that wasn't even my fault. He said, "Well it just went on and on. I didn't know what to say"

So now he was back on my doorstep saying, "When is the skip going and what are you going to do about your dog?" I was so upset since when only the week before his wife had been knocking on the door begging me to let me let her help me with the baby, because they felt guilty about what they had done. I couldn't speak to him. I knew I would just lose my temper so I wrote him a note again, explaining what had happened to me over the past two years. How I was very low and depressed with all the things I had to deal with right now and how the skip and the dog weren't really on my list of priorities and that I would try to keep her quiet and that the skip would go when it was ready as it was parked on a public highway on the street with a permit.

I received a note back the following day saying I was inconsiderate and that actually none of my problems were any of his concern and he didn't believe what I had written anyway. Then I flipped. I don't flip out very often, I don't even know why I wanted to explain myself or why I care why some stupid arrogant neighbour would believe me anyway but I flipped. I went round all my credit card bills all filed neatly in folders, my tablets for my head and knocked on the door to only to have it shut in my face. I even apologised again but then got another letter through my door saying that he was going to report me to the council for nuisance dog barking and what a selfish cow I was.

So the day I flipped I dropped everything. Left the baby with my eldest daughter so he was safe, he had been screaming on and off all day because he was teething. I jumped in the car and drove. I found myself at my local park where I normally went to walk the dog. I'd forgotten how long it had been since I had had the time to walk the dog, and take half an hour for myself. I called up Jamie and told him what had happened, an accumulation of things all getting on top. He always says he is there for me, how much he loves me, but he did what he always does when I most needed him. I was sobbing on the phone and midway through the conversation he said, "I have to go now everyone has just come back home" which meant his wife was back.

It was at that point I picked myself up off the floor again. I realized all these things were happening to me because I was allowing them. I was tired at not being able to say no. I was tired of always playing second best in my relationships. I was worn out paying off the debts and there had to be a better way.

I got a call right out of the blue from a friend that was doing Tantra and energy work. I had taken my boyfriend to see her the year before as a birthday present. It had cost me 400, one of the numerous ways I would spoil him. He was always insistent he had no money even though he lived in a million pound house with no mortgage and I was the one that would always buy lunch even if it were just a Subway sandwich. She asked me how Jamie was and whether he had recovered from his cancer and left his wife. I remember her telling him the day we met that if we spent our lives living in denial all it does it make us sick and we end up dying of some kind of illness. She told him then that we both had a very special bond that would be a crying shame to lose, and wished us well. We had spent the whole day doing the most amazing mind blowing Tantric bodywork and I came away on cloud nine thinking that Jamie had touched my soul. When we came out everything changed there was a call from his wife, nagging because he hadn't answered the phone complaining about some bill. All that feeling was gone so I walked off alone in the park while he chatted to her. It was always like that, if she wasn't calling and nagging he would be telling me how things were with her but he never did anything to leave. I was his safe haven "the Mistress!" in the truest sense. I was just an affair, a secret. Even when he had the cancer, it had been so heart wrenching. I was away in Thailand when he had his operation he had to get one of his friends to text me and tell me it was ok as he wouldn't have his phone on. I'd bought him a lovely present while I was away to cheer him up to come back to nothing.

So things had been hard being the other woman for a year now and Minouska called to see how I was doing in the midst of all my troubles. She asked me to go and work with her. I knew this was the right choice; it would be my saviour from the domination. Instead of spending all my time pushing myself and putting so much creative energy into my work, my website, my films my submissives I could do something proper and go back to what I do best healing people. I told her I had a lot of things on my plate and explained how things were with Jamie and how he was always telling me about his "stuff" with his wife. She said I sense you are just full of shit and actually it makes me feel sick. She didn't mean it in the literal sense I think it was her way of saying get rid of stuff in your life.

I had been thinking about all the things I had made grown men do in the guise of domination. I'd fucked them up the arse with strap ons, teased and denied them until they could no longer control themselves, humiliated them and told them how pathetic they were and not even worthy to lick the shit off my shoes. I'd humiliated them in clubs; I'd forced them to wank in front of me, made them watch while I fucked my boyfriend. Tortured their cocks until their balls turned blue, made them lick my sweaty feet, caned their bottoms till their arse bled. I'd made slaves drink my piss, I'd even made other slaves piss on them, I'd forced slaves to suck and fuck each other. But I realized not one of those things did I ever do without them asking me to do it first. That's what they wanted me to do. It was all about them when in fact they wanted to wrap it all up and say I want to please my mistress.

I admit that sometimes I got off on it; I couldn't have done it for so long if I hadn't. You see a lot of dominatrix who do it for a living because they just want to earn good money; I had invested so much time and effort into my writing, my website, and my films. Everything I did was just a reflection of what I wanted to show about me how I wanted to be the best in what I did, whether it was working in a builder's merchant or running big computer network or being an internationally recognized dominatrix.

But part of the reason I had got into the business was because of my anger and that anger was diminishing each day. There is only so much anger you can carry around and then you have to let it go. I had a client a couple of days before I finally made plans to start winding everything up. He gave me a note. Often slaves did that before a session. It said:

Dear Mistress

Thank you so much for agreeing to see me today. Having seen your website last night I am so excited – especially by your trampling and facesitting. I love a Mistress to be voluptuous and unsquemish, because it means she won't be afraid to us her full weight on me

Just one or two guidelines. First of all I would respectfully ask you not to bruise my face, not to squash or kick me in the balls, and preferably, not to use gags. This session is

INTIMATE ENCOUNTERS

essentially about being UNDERNEATH you. I have driven 270 miles today especially to see you, having already fallen madly in love with you. I have been fantasizing about meeting a cruel death under your stilettos since I saw your picture.

May I respectfully ask you to wear a short mini skirt because I have a fetish for your feet legs and knees and thighs. I would ask that you have as many high heeled shores boots to hand as possible because I would like to be a victim of each.

It went on another page or two……….. then it said I cordially invite you to be an Arrogant Arsehole, Brutal Bitch, Cruel Crushing Cow, Depraved Dominatrix, Heartless Harlot, Vicious Vandal, Laughing Lout, Yeildless Yob, Merciless Monster, Terrifying Torturing Trampler and Extreme Excruciater.

Using Nauseating Nastiness and being Outrageously Obnoxious towards me.

Make me pay for all the men who have messed you about in the past!"

Now there was an offer, I thought to myself, what a shame he wasn't the first client that had come to see me.

Instead I trampled, his face sat on him till he almost passed out and sent him off with such a smile on his face it would probably last for weeks because it was an art and I had learnt it well. And I did actually enjoy it because I orgasmed during the session, but I was thinking more about beating other people up and seeing my boyfriend. And then I thought about Jamie again. I was kinky, well we both were but that's what he loved about me at least I thought. With me he could be himself, he got everything, he could fulfil his sexual fantasies, he could have great vanilla sex whenever he wanted, and I was his best friend to listen to him whenever he needed me. He was always telling me how unhappy he was. But when he was with me Instead of having to look after the kids and do all the cooking and cleaning the house and be nagged, he could come round to me. I'd pay for or cook his favourite lunch. But it's only when you are at the bottom that you can finally start crawling your way back out again. That call I had made, desperate and frantic when I was completely lost and didn't know what to do, made me realize I had to make a choice. I made a decision that night. I sent him a text saying I didn't see any point in seeing him because he could never really be there for me when I needed him because he had a wife. So a couple of weeks later when we had taken a break I sent him this letter:

Dear Jamie

You will be reading this probably after a very lovely day as always. So I don't want you to

INTIMATE ENCOUNTERS

feel sad. Not half as sad as I have felt thinking about writing it. Its Monday 16th so I had already made my decision long before I saw you. I thought if I didn't things would just go on and on and then I would just end up hurting myself more

I have given you until the end of the year to do all the things you said you are going to do. Deadlines are just horrible. The problem is with them is that what happens when you don't meet them. What do I do then? Go into panic mode? Start feeling shit about myself because you haven't left your wife? Start beating myself up all over again? Give you another couple of months? let things drag out for another couple of years? It would all be so simple I guess if I just knew but I don't. For example the one thing I do know is that if I thought you were lying to me about how things were with your wife, that you were sleeping with her and that everything you had ever told me was a pack of lies I would leave. It would all be so easy because then you would be the bad guy and I could blame you and then it would be ok and I could pick myself up off the floor and move on. But your not the bad guy your the good guy. Your the man that makes me feel special whenever your around. You make me smile, you are kind, you are a wonderful lover, and you are there for me most of the time. But when you are always telling me how shit things are, how you are so unhappy in your marriage, how you love me so much and want to leave and I see you do nothing apart from procrastinate and force me into a situation where I push you, then all I do is beat myself up thinking well if you really believed that why would you rather stay there with her than be with me if its so bad. I just end up torturing myself and making myself feel like crap and not worth anything. And that's not what our relationship is supposed to be about. Its supposed to make both of us feeling good about ourselves. I know you keep telling me about how you don't want to leave because of the children but like I have said before if what you say is true its not a healthy relationship for you to be in. You have to want to leave because you want to be happy and for your children as well and not just for me. By me staying with you I am just colluding. Its not healthy for me, not healthy for you, not healthy for your wife and in the long term it will be very unhealthy for your children.

Then the letter went on to say that I was not going to see him again unless he decided he wanted to leave his wife. And finished .....

I have to go on my gut feeling on this one. I just received this in my in box

To be loved like you've never been loved, Rose, you must love like you've never loved.

Sounds pretty easy -
The Universe

INTIMATE ENCOUNTERS

Jamie, I know its hard but we are a mirror of each other, remember I have been where you are already in a different time. I never took the easy route and sometimes harder is better. But you need to be kind to yourself too and only you know how you truly feel and whether you really want to be happy. Today was about us. No pretence, that's who I am, whatever that is, that's all I have to give you, myself. But I cant do that again until your ready to give yourself too. And your not ready to do that because you only do it when it suits you right now. But when you are ready then I will be waiting for you, stronger and happier with no hidden agenda.

I am going to start seeing Jed my counsellor again and try to be strong. Its going to be very hard because I will miss seeing you soooooo much. I will miss making love to you, Speaking to you most days, calling you up telling you what I have been up to and vice versa, planning all kinds of kinky stuff together. I will miss lots. What I wont miss is the emptiness I feel because you are with someone else. But I have to take a chance on what goes around comes around and good things happening to people that are coming from the right place and what's meant to be will be and all that other stuff. So I am going to chuck the ball out into the universe and wait for it to come back when it's ready.

I love you always

Rose Budworth Levine

Rose another dominatrix friend called 'Lola' had written her life story, albeit quite different from mine as she had the cruelest childhood, but there were some similarities. She mentioned that when she became a Dom often the abused becomes the abuser and to some degree that is how I found myself transposing my own abuse by becoming a Dom, except that in terms of abuse, I felt that I was being the abused once again, both in my life as a dominatrix and again as a girlfriend. Jamie was abused, abused by his wife, letting everything around him overtake his own happiness. He had found me, and in some weird way he was the abused. Now without even realizing it, he was abusing me by using me as a dumping ground for his emotional problems with his wife that I was unable to fix. I knew he loved me; it was enough to just keep hoping that one day he might leave. I felt that the only way for our true happiness was to take a chance and let him go and work things out as I had done over the past few years. Our fear of rejection, of being hurt, our fear of change, and our fear of intimacy is what breaks relationships. It also builds them. But its only through our deep and intimate relationship with ourselves that we can really understand ourselves.

Sean called that week to see how his baby was doing. I told him how hard it had been the last few weeks. He had developed a temper and was teething and wanting constant attention. I had split up with my boyfriend, was making daily trips back and forth to my mother cooking and making bottles as my kitchen was still an empty shell being refitted. The house was a mess my life was in chaos. I told him I was tired and worn out and fed up with pretending to be something I was not, hiding my double life from my ten-year-old son, my family, and trying to just please everyone. I explained how my debts were increasing as I was looking after his son rather than working, and told him I had been busy writing. I promised to send him a copy of my book. What a scary thought that was letting my own brother know my most, darkest secrets but then again so would anyone else who ever read it. I promised myself I would give a copy to my counsellor when it was ready. I wondered whether Jamie would be brave enough to leave his wife and thought about the copy of the book I had lent him by Paulo Coelho called the Zahir. I hoped he would understand, and that the penny would drop but then I thought maybe his wife was his Zahir. I wasn't going to beat myself up anymore it was about time I was kind to myself. Then I remembered a friend at college who had given me a certificate he had made for me the day I left with my kids to Canada, to live with my second husband. I had just been through my divorce, fought my Chrohns and taken a chance on finding love again by moving to the other side of the world. It said:

To my dear friend going to Canada
"I don't know many people who actually do what they say. It's a pleasant surprise to know

someone with the courage to do what you're doing on Monday December 4th 2000.

Whether it all works out doesn't matter because you've proven that your word is law. I am proud to know you and have you as my friend. You were the first person I met at college, and I have been getting gifts of friendship ever since.

I truly admire you. You're a great example to all of us and you've inspired me to do the hard things in life not because they're good but because they're the best"

I reminded myself I needed to be my own best friend again.

I guess life is a journey and it takes me back to my favourite comedian bill hicks who said "it's a ride". It's like a roller coaster. Sometimes you just want to get off but if you hold on tight sometimes it's just worth the ride. We have to deal with what life throws at us al the time some people call it shit. I found a profile on informed consent a BDSM website which said:

Taoism : shit happens
Buddhism: if shit happens, it isn't really shit
Islam: if shit happens, it is the will of Allah
Catholicism: if shit happens, you deserve it
Judaism: why does this shit always happen to us?
Atheism: I don't believe this shit

So talking of shit, life never quite turns out as you expect. The day I was about to send my final book off for publishing was also the last day I was to see my boyfriend and give him the letter. But he had had a call the week before to say that his cancer had come back in his throat. From my own experience of dealing with things the only way you can truly be happy is to get rid, and I knew that deep down that why his cancer had come back was because he was deeply unhappy. So I decided in my wisdom instead of abandoning him to desexualize the relationship and be there for him until he could get better and work things through. Celibacy is good for the soul, as I knew from having done it for two years prior to meeting Dan. It's the only way you can really learn about yourself, I believe.

I called up my Tantric advisor Minouska. She thinks that domination is the devils work and explained that I was leaving the business and had plans to learn Tantra and give something back by doing couples therapy. I got a long lecture from her saying that I should stop seeing my boyfriend for six months and leave him to get on and fight his cancer alone. She said his energy was very bad for me and that it was very negative and how my whole life would change if I got rid of him. I thought well that's just fine if you can deal with that but I knew in my own heart if he was to die I would never forgive myself if I never saw him again. Then I smiled when she told me that the work she did was special and how I would never be able to feel good about myself doing domination. And suggested I started doing sensual massage on men to make myself feel better. I didn't need to make myself feel better, I knew what the answers was and massaging men and their egos certainly wasn't that. So what my future is now who knows?

I didn't write my story for people to judge me or feel sorry for me. I remember speaking to my publisher and saying how I was so concerned about people finding out who I was. I am not ashamed of anything I have done in my life but was concerned that I was coming from the right place. I just wrote for me and perhaps it might help other people along the way. What people may think of me is their own choice, I am just telling it how it was for me. I have dealt with all kinds of shit most of my life, some of it my making, some of it not. I guess only time will tell what shit comes up next, whatever category or belief my shit fits into at least it will be an interesting read.

I received a call from my publisher about a week before finishing my book, he asked me if I had decided what picture I wanted on the book as I had decided to remain anonymous. I have a chest in my lounge full of pictures from my childhood; I remember having a happy childhood until I reached puberty because I was innocent. I wasn't aware of my mother and fathers affairs I was a carefree girl that wandered around the streets hanging off my eldest Sean's arms, knickers half falling down playing in the sunshine looking up to my brother as if he was the best brother in the world. I have that photograph in my head for years but the innocent went a long time ago. I thought about Sean, how he had made a mess of relationships too, his two failed marriages, and his last one about to be finished. His gorgeous baby boy chuckling to himself as my daughter Emma played with him kissing his feet and blowing raspberries on his belly. I thought about how difficult things would be for him when he finally came over to look after his son as a single father. I realized I had lost all my innocence a long time ago. I couldn't remember the last time I was happy and it made me cry.

I called my closest confidents and friends, Pasquale, an Italian I had made friends with through the domination. He had been there for me on so many occasions and helped me to be strong. I told him how I had made a decision to end my relationship until my boyfriend was ready to come back. How I had picked myself up off the floor again and he said "you know what, I am proud of you mate, your doing ok, you're a survivor". I said to him "you know I hate that, that's what everyone has called me all of my life - a survivor and it makes me sound like a victim - but you know what I don't want to just survive anymore, I want to live". So now my journey really begins.

I saw him again yesterday and explained that I had had to bend the rules a bit because of Jamie's cancer, and we chatted and talked and laughed and he told me how crazy and impatient I was. He said he would have to be a chaperone for me each time Jamie and I met up in case the pair of us tried any funny business. I told him how much I'd miss him when he went to Thailand and on the drive home in the car when I finally had time to compose my thoughts I turned the music up loud, some nice trippy dance music that would let my mind wander for a few brief moments and I remembered Bill Hills again and yes life is just a ride, I guess I'll have to ride this one out and see what happens.

11- DIAMONDS ARE FOREVER

I woke up one morning around 5 am. I had fed the baby, made myself the usual ritualistic cup of tea and a cigarette. I had arranged to go and see a therapist who did a technique called "the journey". It seemed pretty apt with the old Bill Hicks theme running through my life, about my life being a roller coaster with all its ups and downs. I was a little nervous that morning and it often affected my stomach.

The baby was now happily playing in his cot. While sitting in the loo contemplating my day ahead, I had a million and one things to do. I had to drop the baby at my mothers for the day. Drive over to Cambridge and then on my way back I had banking and other boring stuff to do. My thoughts were drifting when suddenly this "thought" just popped in my head, as I was about to have a dump! Oh my God I thought. It's not true, it can't be. I tried to rationalise it and the more I did the more upset and anxious I got and the more I started to panic and cry. Its not the first time this particular thought had popped into my head before, although one day before my 45th birthday, while I was about to have a dump, seemed like an odd day for it to rear its ugly head again.

I think I had been crying for about an hour before I arrived at my Mums, baby in-hand looking totally dishevelled. She said "Oh my god what's the matter". Then I tried to explain. In the past, namely during rights of passage such as puberty I have had odd memories about my childhood that I couldn't recall. I used to have recurring nightmares about being pinned down by a dark stranger. When I reached puberty I was very body conscious and wouldn't let my father see me in my underwear. I always put it down to just being a teenager but I didn't like to be held close by him either. Then again when I had my first child I had this totally irrational fear when she was first born that my father would abuse her and found it very uncomfortable watching him hold her as a small baby. My father wouldn't hurt a fly and he was great with children so I had always pushed my irrational fears to the back of my mind. The thought that he could have ever sexually abused me abhorred me and I would feel sick to the core. Then I had heard stories about abuse in the family of other people but none of them had anything to do with my father.

So this "thought" or should I say an image or memory of my childhood that appeared that morning was not of my father. It was of my grandfather. So when I arrived at my mums and explained everything, of course she was very shocked, but surprisingly she didn't question me or say it's all your imagination. "She said you know why you have struggled all these years Rose? Because your grandfather was the spitting image of your dad"

It all started to make sense and everything seemed to fit into place. Like a jigsaw puzzle. Like that small piece I had been looking for, for the last forty or so years were finally found. My mind was

INTIMATE ENCOUNTERS

racing! OK I thought so what am I supposed to do with my jigsaw puzzle now? Stick it together with cellotape and put it on the wall, chuck in the bin or give it to the charity shop so some other person can put it all back together again. I didn't really now how I felt at that point. I did know a few things about my grandfather and that was he was a nasty piece of work. In a later conversation with my stepmother who knew him well. I told her what had happened and the first thing she said was she thought that he had been abusing my auntie for years and possibly my cousin too. I had no idea where I was going to take this. Raking it up with my dad wouldn't do any good. He hated his father, so much so he and his brother went to his grave and told him what a useless bastard he was when he was buried.

I thought the best thing to do was to let my feelings out, and boy did I! I cried for ten days pretty much non-stop from the moment I woke up, till the minute I went to bed. I couldn't stop crying. I thought I was going to drown in my own tears. Then I woke up one day and felt like it all seemed a bit better.

The older we get the faster our lives seem to move. Sometimes at such an ever-increasing rate we look back and just don't know where the days have gone. I had done "the journey" that day which helped a little but my days are very up and down now. It's now three months passed and I have sold the property I was renovating to pay off all my debts. My brother Sean is now living with me looking after the baby. I speak to the boyfriend from time to time. I had still have not slept with him, and he is still promising to leave his wife. I am keeping myself busy setting up my therapy business, have myself booked on a number of courses and working through the transition of stopping domination.

My health is deteriorating again. I am on the menopausal change. I seem to be permanently on my period all the time now. Life feels like a bit of a struggle. Sometimes I feel that things were better when they were left hidden and I didn't remember. It's a bit like the reference Brandon Bays makes in her opening statement on her book the Journey about everyone being like a diamond when they are born. Bright and pure and that its years of muck and dirt that we use to cover up who we are, including copious amounts of nail polish until we have no idea what we are anymore. Then we have to uncover all the muck and dirt to find the diamond again. I wrote a poem for my boyfriend a couple of months ago thinking I might help him.

It's another year on and our dreams are all shattered

All that we hoped for and all that had mattered

My eyes are still sore from crying rose coloured tears

You now face your own demons as I have faced my own fears

That cancer is a fucker it will keep on returning

INTIMATE ENCOUNTERS

If you don't pull out its root that lies in your heart yearning

I'm not talking about me or some lover or wife

I am talking about you, what you want in your life

It's much easier to forget to just get on and do

Numbs the brain and the senses and our soul too

So I found you a mirror that was special and good

It was tucked in the cellar and carved in oak wood

It's been hidden for years in a dusty old room

It holds answers to secrets you never dreamed could

When you look in the mirror, what can you see?

Is it you, or you children, your wife, or me?

I think none of the above because the view isn't clear

It's just smeared with anger and guilt and fear

Pull the cloth from your pocket and start to erase

All the smears on the mirror and start clearing the haze

As you wipe away layers of dirt built over time

You will fight back the tears as you clean off the grime

Your fingers are hurting your cant rub anymore

You'll leave it for now there's a knock at the door

Oh I'll deal with it later you say to yourself

Rose Budworth Levine

No one cares about that old mirror put it back on the shelf

But you can't do that Jamie its too special to leave

The woods starting to rot and it needs air to breathe

The mirror is tarnished you must do it in time

It takes forever to polish and bring back the shine

Then you will look in the mirror it will all become clear

With each rub of the cloth you have faced all your fear

As you look in the mirror you see only YOU

No kids, no lover, no wife - My god what will you do?

Say hello to yourself for the first time in years

Do not mess up the mirror again with your tears

It's a special mirror that needs nurture and care like you

If you look after it well it will be honest and true

It will reflect all your dreams, your hopes and your fears

But the maintenance polish is not your own tears

It's only small Jamie not much bigger than a locket

If you keep it with you always, it will fit in your pocket

INTIMATE ENCOUNTERS

Just remember to look after it as I try to do

And it will always be kind to you and let you be YOU.

I always seem to be helping people in one way or another. Helping them out and "Dealing with their shit". I had a fall out with my good friend Pasquale over someone who had been staying with me. I was trying to help out as usual. He wrote me and told me that he thought I spent my time dealing with everyone else's problems because I couldn't face mine. I thought he was probably right and that. I think it's about time I started taking my own advice.

Sexual abuse causes all kinds of hurt and anger and fear. My boyfriend was sexually abused too. I guess that's why we have such a strong connection. I just didn't realise I was too. For this little girl that liked to go in all the closets and find out what she was getting for Christmas every year and never liked any kind of surprises I did a really good job of covering this little cracker up for the last 40 or so years.

I read some interesting research on the Internet about Disassociation Identity syndrome or Multiple Personality Disorder or MPD for short and how it develops in severely abused children. They learn to "cover up" as a coping mechanism. The more severe the abuse the more personalities I develop. I have to say I did find it very ironic because the initials MPD are what my submissives call me for short. Luckily I only have one personality well maybe two, but then again don't we all.

It's Saturday 29th October 2007 and I am sitting outside a coffee shop killing time waiting for my train back to Bedford. I have just been on a refresher course for my therapy work. It was almost seven years to the day that I left my so called comfortable life with my husband and started afresh with my children.

Life has taken the most unexpected turn of events for the last few years. As I stir my coffee glancing at the passers by I see a young man walking up the street towards me. He has long floppy hair, casual dress, headphones on carrying a rucksack. I have to second glance for a moment. It looks like Dan. He walks past me with the kind of carefree attitude I loved. For a moment I think about Dan that innocent smile, and how I felt when I watched him killing himself with the alcohol. I wonder how he is doing and think of him working in the record shop with me as just a distant memory.

I remind myself that I have my whole life ahead of me. I am forty five and I feel like I have lived a roller coaster life of a thousand dreams, untold nightmares and unfulfilled wishes but I feel like I am about to start on a new journey. There have been days when I have wanted to get off this ride but in this moment, I remind myself not to be so hard on myself and that I have come a long way. I remind myself life is not so bad. I remind myself of all the debts I have cleared, all the challenges I have faced and overcome and the earlier lunch conversation I had with the other students reminds me that I am going to be in Thailand at Christmas for two whole months. I realise that there is no such thing as coincidence or serendipity and I smile to myself and that if it wasn't for all the things that had happened to me both good and bad I wouldn't be the person I was today, sitting here enjoying this moment.

I grab my coat and walk towards the train station. Perfect timing there is a train waiting for me at the platform. I remind myself of all the promises the broken promises and all the promises I made to myself and make a mental note to post a copy of my book to Dan. He loved to read books and said that when he had finished reading a book he would leave it somewhere, usually on a train so that someone else would pick it up and read it. He said books where like birds their pages represented the wings and they had a freedom all of their own. I wondered whether he would read it or leave it on the train for someone else to read.

I start to laugh to myself. With the image of my friend saying to me "It's a funny old life". Perhaps I was mad after all. I guess I will figure it all out in the end. I suppose I need to fish around and find that diamond again and give it a good old polish. I am sure its hiding somewhere.

.

THE END

www.ingramcontent.com/pod-product-compliance
Lightning Source LLC
Chambersburg PA
CBHW030933090426
42737CB00007B/405